Nutrition Essentials
Third Edition

A Guidebook for the Fitness Professional

Joe Cannon, MS

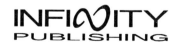

INFI∞ITY
PUBLISHING

Joe Cannon's Website: www.Joe-Cannon.com

ISBN 978-0-7414-1892-0

Published by:

INFIᗯITY
PUBLISHING

INFINITY PUBLISHING
1094 New DeHaven Street, Suite 100
West Conshohocken, PA 19428-2713
Toll-free (877) BUY BOOK
Local Phone (610) 941-9999
Fax (610) 941-9959
Info@buybooksontheweb.com
www.buybooksontheweb.com

Printed in the United States of America
Published October 2012

Table of Contents

For Mom & Dad

May there be libraries in heaven…

Acknowledgments

I have always felt that we are truly blessed by the quality of the people that we can count among our friends. I have been blessed by some friends who I would like to formally thank now, who assisted me in various capacities during the creation of this book.

Much thanks also to Kelly Bixler and Dianna Mills, MS who were instrumental in sharing both their unique insights and editing skills.

Thanks Bill Leinhauser, Timothy DiFelice and Adam Freedman for their continued encouragement, reassurance and friendship over the years.

I also would like to thank everyone who is an owner of previous editions of *Nutrition Essentials*. Your faith in me as a writer and educator have been an inspiration and were the key influences in my decision refine this book to further meet your needs.

What's This Book About?

With the first edition of Nutrition Essentials, I began my quest to bring to the fitness professional a resource where he or she could read concise and up to date information on a myriad of nutrition and fitness-related topics and issues which they will likely encounter over the course of their career. This book, builds upon the previous editions by providing additional information to help broaden the knowledge of readers.

As always, I had two main goals when writing this book. First, I wanted to create a text that would help fitness professionals cut through the sometimes murky and complicated waters that seem to permeate our field. Second, I wanted to present a text which explained complex topics in easy to understand language. It's likely that many of you have a large library of wellness-related books. Some of those books however explain things in complex and technical language. Nutrition Essentials was written to help bridge that gap and foster greater understanding on the part of the reader. This can be particularly invaluable for those studying for a certification and want answers fast.

Every chapter is independent of the others so readers can start anywhere he or she desires. I have also included a glossary of terms at the end of the book to further assist with researching and understanding the major topics presented in the text. In addition a detailed index is included to help people quickly jump to the area they are looking for.

It is my hope that you will find Nutrition Essentials of value. As before, comments on this book are always welcome. Readers are encouraged to visit my website, www.Joe-Cannon.com to share with me their thoughts and impressions about this book. There you will also find a wealth of other information which, I hope you will enjoy.

Joe Cannon

Chapter 1

The Macronutrients

The term "macro" means *big*. Macronutrients are molecules which we can obtain energy from and which are also nutritious, providing vitamins, minerals, fiber and other important factors needed for optimal health. Macronutrients are also consumed in greater quantities than other nutrients. There are three macronutrients: *carbohydrates*, *fats* and *proteins*. Below is a brief review of the macronutrients, along with other relevant topics that fitness professionals should be familiar with.

Carbohydrate

The term carbohydrate is another name for sugar. Carbohydrates ("carbs") are called carbohydrates because they all contain the elements carbon, hydrogen and oxygen.[36] Examples of carbohydrates include bread, rice, potatoes, glucose (blood sugar), lactose (milk sugar), broccoli and other vegetables. Most carbohydrates for the human diet are derived from plants.[36] Carbohydrates can be subdivided into the following types of molecules: monosaccharides, disaccharides, oligosaccharides and polysaccharides. Each name is related to the number of sugars that make up the molecule in question. For example, monosaccharides are single sugar molecules while disaccharides are composed of two sugar molecules linked together. Polysaccharides are composed of many (usually from ten to thousands) of sugar molecules.

Polysaccharides

Polysaccharides are composed of between ten to literally thousands of sugar molecules chemically bonded together. Examples of polysaccharides include starch, glycogen and fiber, to name a few.

- **Starch.** Starch is the carbohydrate storage molecule of plants. Starch is found in foods such as spaghetti, rice, cereal and bread.

- **Glycogen.** Glycogen forms the stored sugar reserves in animals and humans. Glycogen is found in both the muscle—where it serves as a direct energy source to the muscles during activity—and the liver, where it allows for an even distribution of blood sugar levels between meals. Glycogen is produced from the bonding together of many glucose molecules during the process called *glucogenesis* and broken down by the process called *glycogenolysis* [36]. Thus, glucose and glycogen are essentially the same thing, just different forms of the

7

same molecule. As will be discussed later, glycogen breakdown, along with fats, serve as the major nutrients used as fuel during aerobic exercise. Glycogen is often called the *limiting factor* because when one runs out of glycogen, exercise stops. Runners sometime call this phenomenon "hitting the wall". The average person has between 1500 to 2000 calories of glycogen stored in his or her body. This is enough energy to power a 20 mile run at high speed.[36]

Fiber

Fiber is a general term used to describe indigestible plant structures.[26] Fiber is found only in plants.[37] Fiber gives "bulk" to food and helps people feel full. In terms of weight control, fiber may aid in reducing weight gain and obesity by reducing the number of calories consumed. While the typical American roughly contains 12-15 grams of fiber per day from their diet the recommended dietary allowance (RDA) for fiber is 25-35 grams per day.[26] Fiber can be divided into both water-soluble fiber and water-insoluble fiber. Studies show that water-soluble fiber such as pectin and oats can modestly reduce blood cholesterol levels.[26] Water-insoluble fiber does not have cholesterol lowering effects but may offer other healthy bennefits.[36] In addition to evidence linking increased fiber intake to reduced obesity and cholesterol levels, fiber also contains other nutrients beneficial to health. For example, fiber contains magnesium which may play a role in reducing diabetes.[26] Examples of high fiber foods include Fiber One cereal, Raisin Bran cereal, whole wheat pasta, brown rice and oatmeal. Vegetables are also rich in fiber and is one of the reasons nutrition professionals usually counsel people to increase their intake of these foods.

Fiber and Health

Dietary fiber has received much attention as of late because of research showing that enhanced fiber intake is associated with reduced risk of various diseases. Studies of large numbers of people (epidemiological studies) have shown that people who consume the most fiber tend to have reduced risks for diabetes, obesity, heart disease, high blood pressure, and intestinal disorders.[46, 47] Theories abound as to how fiber-rich diets protect us from these disorders. Some of those theories include (1) that added fiber may decrease the amount of time that harmful materials are in the body, (2) that fiber dilutes and/or binds harmful materials, reducing the chance that they cause problems in the body and (3) that fiber may result in a scraping or scrubbing action on the cells of the gastrointestinal tract, which in theory would dislodge harmful substances, preventing them from doing harm.[36] It may be that fiber exerts all of these functions as well as others which have yet to be determined.

Throughout the world, carbohydrate serves as a major component of daily calorie intake. In the typical American diet, carbohydrates make up between 40-50% of daily calories.[36] Some experts recommend that individuals who exercise should increase their carbohydrate intake to 60% of daily calories.[36] All carbohydrates are not created equal however, a fact that seems to have been missed by many. Carbohydrates from cookies, cakes and other snack foods are not the same as complex carbohydrates from vegetables and whole grains. Complex carbohydrates, like those from fruits and vegetables, tend to not only contain fewer calories but also are generally rich in vitamins, minerals, fiber and the popular phytonutrients that are often talked about in the news today. Thus, where possible, people should strive to improve intake of complex carbohydrates like those found in fruits and vegetables and limit those derived from candy, soda, cookies or cakes.

Lactose Intolerance

Some people do not have the ability to digest milk sugar (lactose). Specifically, these individuals lack an enzyme called *lactase* which breaks down lactose. For the person with lactose intolerance, consumption of milk or milk products which contain lactose may result in cramping and other gastrointestinal distresses. Over-the-counter products and lactose free foods are available to help these individuals eat a healthy diet.

Carbohydrates and Exercise

As was mentioned previously, carbohydrates are essential to the exercising individual because they are a rate-limiting fuel. That is, once carbohydrates are depleted from the body, exercise performance decreases dramatically. More specifically, nobody wins a marathon on a low-carbohydrate diet.

Carbohydrates are used in greater amounts as exercise intensity increases.[36] Stated another way, carbohydrate burning is increased during activities that are of *high intensity and short duration*. The greater the need for quick energy, the greater the demand is placed on carbohydrates for fuel. For example, running a 5 minute mile uses a greater percentage of carbohydrates than running a 15 minute mile.

Carbohydrates and Ketones

Carbohydrates are essential to the burning of fat. The reason for this is that metabolic byproducts from carbohydrate metabolism are needed to properly break down body fat.[36] This also ramps up protein breakdown as well (carbs reduce protein breakdown). In the absence of carbs the body also steps up its production of ketones. Ketones are normally made in small amounts but are increased during low carb diets. In the absence of carbs, the body can use ketones for fuel - but at a price. Because they are acidic in nature, prolonged elevated ketones (*ketosis*) could, in theory be fatal especially in those with pre-existing medical issues.

Fat

The energy stored within the fat reserves, represent the most abundant source of energy in the body.[36] For example, the average adult male has between 50,000 and 100,000 calories of energy stored as fat.[36]

Another name for fat is *lipid*. Thus, fats and lipids are sometimes used interchangeably. At the molecular level, fats basically look like long chains of carbon atoms surrounded by hydrogen atoms. Contrary to what some may think, fats, serve a variety of important functions in the body. Just some of the functions of fats include making up key cellular components of every cell membrane of the body, insulation of the body to cold temperatures, shock absorption for crucial organs and forming components of a wide variety of molecules indispensable to the proper functioning of the body. Fat is also a good source of energy with each gram of fat containing nine calories. While this may not seem like a lot, consider that the body fat of an average person could supply enough energy to run non-stop for about 120 hours.[36] Because of the role that fats play in diseases and syndromes ranging from heart disease and some forms of cancer to diabetes and obesity to name a few, several experts recommend that Americans consume no more than 30 percent of daily calories from fat.

Aside from being the long-term energy storage molecule of the body, fat also constitutes a major source of calories during long-duration exercise, like running a marathon. While fat mobilization begins almost as soon as exercise begins, it does not represent a major contributor to our energy needs at the start of exercise. As exercise continues however, the amount of fat used increases. Another way of saying this is that fat is used significantly as a fuel source during any activity that is of *low intensity and long duration*.

Calories of the Macronutrients	
Macronutrient	**Calorie per gram**
• Carbohydrate	4
• Protein	4
• Fat	9

The table above provides a quick overview of the calories contained in each of the macronutrients. As can be seen, both carbohydrate and protein each contain 4 calories per gram. Fat, on the other hand, contains 9 calories per gram. Looking at this from another point of view, if they both weighted the same, fat would have 2 ½ times the calories of either carbohydrate or protein. This fact has profound implications on weight loss. Stated another way, reducing fat from the diet, also reduces a lot of calories—and reductions in calories are the key to weight loss.

Triglycerides

Triglyceride is yet another name for fat. Triglycerides are not only the most abundant fat in the body,[36] but also represent our major storage form of fat. Triglycerides are stored within specialized cells called *adipose cells* or fat cells.

Saturated vs. Unsaturated Fats

As stated previously, fats essentially look like long chains of carbon atoms surrounded by hydrogen atoms. The number of hydrogen atoms which surround the carbon chain of fats gives rise to the terms saturated fats and unsaturated fats. *Saturated fats* are literally saturated with hydrogen atoms. In other words, with saturated fats, every available attachment point on the carbon chain is occupied with a hydrogen atom. This alters the chemical properties of the fat. Research has linked diets high in saturated fats as a contributing factor to heart disease. While animal products like beef, and some dairy products tend to be high in saturated fat, so too can some foods derived from plants [36]. For example, coconut and palm oils tend to be high in saturated fat.[36] Cookies, cakes, pies and similar commercially produced items are also a source of saturated fats. On food labels, saturated fats may not be listed as "saturated fat". Rather, they may be identified by two alternate names—*hydrogenated* or *partially hydrogenated* oils. Generally, saturated fats are usually easily recognized because they are solid at room temperature. Experts recommend that people eat no more than 10 percent of daily calories from saturated fat.[36]

Unsaturated fats are said to be more "heart healthy" than saturated fats. As a general rule, unsaturated fats are obtained from plant–based foods and are usually recognized as being liquid at room temperature. It is important to remember, however, that both saturated and unsaturated fats each have nine calories per gram. Unsaturated fats can be further sub-divided according to their degree of saturation with hydrogen. For example, an unsaturated fat that has one space available that is not occupied by a hydrogen atom is called *monounsaturated*. An unsaturated fat that has many spaces available that are not occupied by hydrogen atoms is termed *polyunsaturated*.

Food Sources of Fats	
Type of Fat	**Sources**
• Saturated Fat	butter, whole milk, coconut oil, palm oil
• Polyunsaturated Fat	evening primrose oil, flaxseed, tuna, safflower oil
• Monounsaturated Fat	peanuts, olive oil, canola oil

What are Trans Fatty Acids?

Trans fatty acids have a different molecular arrangement of atoms than do saturated or unsaturated fats. Trans fatty acids are formed during *hydrogenation*—the process of making saturated fats. Thus they tend to be found in processed foods like cakes, cookies and fried foods. Some studies have shown that trans fats can reduce good cholesterol (HDL), and raise bad cholesterol (LDL).[51] This means trans fats might increase the risk for of heart disease. Other research has noted that women whose bodies contain high levels of trans fatty acids are about 40% more likely to develop breast cancer than women with lower levels of trans fatty acids.[36] Preliminary research stemming mostly from laboratory animals hints that diets high in trans fats may reduce testosterone levels.[68] The implications for this on exercising humans requires further study. The role that trans fatty acids play in disease is still being debated. Identifying foods that contain these fats is relatively easy. Foods whose labels use the terms hydrogenated or partially hydrogenated tend to contain trans fats. Thus, limiting hydrogenated and partially hydrogenated fats also limits trans fats. Because of the link to cancer and heart disease, food labels in the U.S. now list trans fats.

Cholesterol

Cholesterol is a lipid that is only found in animal tissues.[36] In humans, cholesterol can be obtained either by eating cholesterol-containing foods or by being made naturally in the liver. Contrary to what some may have been told in the past, cholesterol serves several very important functions. For example, cholesterol is a component of every cell membrane in the human body, helping cells to maintain integrity. If it were not for cholesterol, life on earth might not have arisen. In addition, cholesterol is integral to the production of testosterone, estrogen and vitamin D. If it were not for cholesterol, these compounds might not exist.

In spite of its crucial role in health, too much cholesterol can be a health problem. Because the risk of heart disease tends to increase as blood cholesterol concentrations increase, experts recommend maintaining a relatively low total cholesterol level, preferably less than 200 milligrams per deciliter. Sometimes those with high cholesterol levels try to control it by eating less cholesterol-containing foods. Because the body also makes cholesterol, this strategy may or may not work. It's possible that the body may compensate for this by making more cholesterol.

Those who have elevated blood cholesterol are advised to work with their physician to attempt to reduce levels, given the positive health effects gained from lowering this lipid. For example, a one percent reduction in cholesterol levels reduces heart disease risk by two percent.[36] Besides cholesterol itself, two types of cholesterol – HDL and LDL – are also important for overall heart health. HDL and LDL are the so-called *good* and *bad* cholesterol respectively. Let's review each briefly here and describe what it does.

- **HDL.** HDL stands for *high density lipoprotein*. HDL transports excess cholesterol back to the liver where it is recycled. HDL is commonly referred to as "good" cholesterol because it removes excess cholesterol from the bloodstream, reducing its potential to be incorporated into artery-clogging plaque. It is recommended that on blood tests, HDL levels be greater than or equal to 40 mg/dl. An HDL level of 60 or better is considered a *negative* risk *factor* for heart disease.[2] This means that excess cholesterol is cleared from the blood so efficiently that the chances of it building up are very low. Studies show that exercise (especially aerobic exercise) can raise HDL levels in many individuals.

- **LDL.** LDL stands for *low density lipoprotein* and is the so-called "bad" cholesterol. LDL transports cholesterol from the liver where it is made, to the cells of the body which use the cholesterol in a variety of ways (like making testosterone and vitamin D for example). Because high blood cholesterol levels are associated with heart disease, elevated levels of LDL may theoretically transport more cholesterol than is needed. This may result in cholesterol building up in blood vessels, resulting in the formation of artery-clogging plaque. On blood tests, LDL should be less than 100 milligrams per deciliter (mg/dl). Studies show that exercise – especially aerobic exercise – may lower LDL in some individuals.

Accepted Blood Lipid Levels	
Lipid	**Accepted Level (mg/dl)**
Cholesterol	Less than 200
HDL	Greater than 40
LDL	Less than 100
Triglycerides	Less than 150

What About The Cholesterol Ratios?

When cholesterol is checked by a doctor, one of the calculations that is usually performed is the *total cholesterol / HDL ratio*. This is sometimes abbreviated as *CHOL / HDL risk ratio*. This number calculated by dividing the total cholesterol by the HDL. For example, if your total cholesterol was 150 mg/dl and HDL level was 60 mg/dl, the ratio would be 150 ÷ 60 = 2.5. There is a relationship between the risk of having a heart attack or stroke and the Chol/HDL risk ratio. When interpreting this number, the goal is to keep the ratio below 5. For every full number decrease in this ratio (for example going from 5 to 4) the risk of heart disease drops by 50 percent.[38]

Another ratio you are likely to see is the *LDL / HDL ratio*. This number tells how much LDL is present in relation to how much HDL is in the blood. It is calculated by dividing the LDL number by the HDL number. Low risk is between 0.5 to 3.0. High risk is 6.0 or more.

Protein

Aside from being one of the main constituents of muscle tissue, protein forms a wide variety of molecules in the body. Some have estimated that proteins comprise over 50,000 different compounds in the human body.[36] The individual properties of each of these protein-containing structures are determined by the sequence of amino acids – the building blocks of proteins. Humans require 20 different amino acids to make all of the different protein structures found in the body. By changing the order or arrangement of amino acids, it is possible to make different proteins which serve different functions and have different properties. This is similar to how words are formed. For example, there are 26 letters in the English alphabet. Yet these 26 letters can form hundreds of thousands of words. Different arrangements of letters make different words, just as different arrangements of amino acids make different proteins. Good sources of proteins include chicken, turkey, whey, soy, beef and tuna to name a few. The amino acids that make up proteins can be further broken down into essential amino acids and non-essential amino acids, which are discussed below.

Essential & Non-Essential Amino Acids

Amino acids are usually classified as being either essential or non-essential. Essential amino acids are those that must be obtained from eating food or using supplements. The non-essential amino acids are those which the body can make and thus do not have to be obtained from the diet. Non-essential amino acids are not less essential than essential amino acids; rather they are called non-essential only because our bodies have the ability to make them from other foods that we eat. The table below list the different essential and non-essential amino acids.

Essential & Non-Essential Amino Acids

Essential Amino Acids		Non-Essential Amino Acids	
• Tryptophan	• Leucine	• Glycine	• Cystine
• Valine	• Lysine	• Arginine	• Proline
•Threonine	• Phenylalanine	• Glutamic Acid	• Aspartic Acid
• Isoleucine	• Methionine	• Glutamine	• Serine
	• Histidine	• Alanine	• Tyrosine
			• Asparagine

The task of memorizing the amino acids as well as trying to remember which is essential and non-essential has probably kept more than one student awake at night. One easy way to remember the amino acids as well as those that are essential and non-essential is to assign a phrase to them that helps jog your memory. Take the essential amino acids for example. Starting at tryptophan and reading down, gives the letters 'TV TILL PM". Each letter represents a different essential amino acid. Thus, TV TILL PM is one way people can use to help remember the essential amino acids. Histidine is usually left out of the list of essential amino acids. Histidine is unique because it is controversial whether or not it is essential in adults.

The same memory-jogging technique can be applied to the non-essential amino acids. Starting at glycine and reading down yields "GAGG AC PASTA" Thus, GAGG AC PASTA is a way to help people remember the non-essential amino acids.

One issue that often confuses people with respect to non-essential amino acids is that the classification as "non-essential" gives the impression that because they are made in the body, that they serve no "essential" role. Ongoing research however is finding that nothing can be farther from the truth. Research is uncovering that individual non-essential amino acids may, under some circumstances be essential. This has given rise to the term "conditionally essential" amino acid. In other words, under some circumstances or conditions, an amino acid that normally is made in sufficient amounts, might not be enough to meet the body's needs. In these situations, supplementation may be needed. One example of this is the amino acid glutamine. While normally considered a non-essential amino acid, some research finds that the body's need for glutamine may increase following surgery or disease.[66] Another example is histidine, which is essential in infants but may or may not be in adults. Some speculate that histidine may affect the immune system although this is controversial. Yet another example of a conditionally essential amino acid is arginine, where increased consumption may benefit people undergoing trauma such as surgery or severe burns.[67]

Nitrogen Balance

The phrase *nitrogen balance* refers to a situation where protein intake equals protein excretion or loss from the body. When protein intake equals protein loss, the body is said to be in a state of balance or homeostasis. A *positive* nitrogen balance occurs when protein intake exceeds protein excretion. Situations such as pregnancy, childhood and participating in a resistance training program all lead to a positive nitrogen balance.[36] A *negative* nitrogen balance, on the other hand, occurs when protein excretion exceeds protein intake. This situation may occur when the body breaks down its own protein because of inadequate calories. A negative nitrogen balance might be expected to occur in those suffering from long-term illness, such as cancer or anorexia. It can also occur in senior citizens who do not exercise or eat well. It is important to note that a negative nitrogen balance can occur even when protein intake is adequate or when it exceeds the recommended dietary allowance.[36] Inadequate calorie intake is the most important factor contributing to a negative nitrogen balance.

Protein & Weight Loss

Some people attempting to reduce body weight may increase the amount of protein they consume. It turns out, there may be something to this tactic. Protein can stimulate metabolism, the speed that calories are burned. Thus, the addition of protein-containing meals to one's daily regimen might help foster weight loss. Protein also speeds water loss which can also help lower body weight, albeit temporarily. Given that dieting may increase protein breakdown, the addition of protein foods to the diet may in theory also spare body proteins from being catabolized. The calculation of how much protein is needed by adults will be addressed in a separate chapter.

Macronutrient Determination

Sometimes, the fitness professional may wish to show clients how to calculate the number of grams of carbohydrate, fat and protein that are in a diet. This is handy for those who do not wish to count calories but would rather focus on counting grams. For example, someone on a particular diet may be instructed to eat 190 grams of carbohydrates to maintain their dietary regimen. To illustrate this, let's use the following scenario. Suppose someone were eating a diet that consisted of the following:
A diet of 1800 total calories a day consisting of:

> 60% carbohydrate
> 15% protein
> 25% fat

From these, determine the number of grams of carbohydrate, protein and fat that this diet is composed of.

> **Determine the number of grams of carbohydrate:**
> 1800 total calories X 0.6 = 1080 calories from carbohydrates
> 1080 ÷ 4 calories per gram = **270 grams of carbohydrates**
>
> **Determine the number of grams of protein:**
> 1800 total calories X 0.15 = 270 calories from protein
> 270 ÷ 4 calories per gram = **68 grams of protein**
>
> **Determine the number of grams of fat:**
> 1800 total calories x 0.25 = 450 calories from fat
> 450 ÷ 9 calories per gram = **50 g from fat**

So, this hypothetical 1800 calorie diet that is 60% carbs, 15% protein and 25% fat is composed of 270 grams of carbs, 68 grams of protein and 50 grams of fat.

Some may be wondering where the numbers *0.6, .15* and *.25* came from. These are decimal equivalents of 60%, 15% and 25% for carb, protein and fat respectively. Converting any number from a percent to a decimal is simply a matter of moving the decimal point two places to the left. Thus:

- 60% = 0.6
- 15% = 0.15
- 25% = 0.25

Chapter 2

Energy & How We Make it

What is Energy?

Energy is usually defined as the ability to do work. Work can be anything from reading these words, walking the dog, working out or even keeping your heart beating. It all requires energy. We obtain energy from the foods we eat, specifically the proteins, carbs and fats described in the last chapter. Let's now discuss how we use the energy in food to make the type of energy that our body's need.

The Energy Contained in Food

The energy contained within food is measured in calories. A calorie is a unit of heat energy. Specifically, a calorie is the amount of heat needed to raise one kilogram (i.e. one liter) of water one degree Celsius. This definition gives rise to the alternative name for calories – *kilogram calories* or *K calories* for short. Humans derive calories from the *macronutrients* – protein, fat and carbohydrate. The amount of calories contained in protein, fat and carbohydrate is known. As was mentioned previously, every gram of protein and carbohydrate contains 4 calories. Every gram of fat contains 9 calories. A concept that is not often talked about however is that before we can use these calories, they must first be transformed into a type of energy that our bodies understand how to use. For you and I and everybody else on earth, ultimately, this form of energy is a molecule called ATP, which will now be discussed.

What is ATP?

Humans, like all living things, must consume food to survive. Most people know that we use the energy contained within food to provide us with the energy to exercise and carry out our daily activities. What some may not be aware of however is that the energy contained within food is not immediately available to us. In other words, the energy stored within the chemical bonds that hold the atoms of food together must be rearranged into a form of energy that we can use. For humans, that usable form of energy is stored in a molecule called *adenosine triphosphate* (ATP for short).

ATP is the ultimate energy molecule that we use to power all of our activities. ATP consists of a molecule of adenosine, chemically bonded to three phosphate atoms. There is a lot energy contained within the chemical bond holding the third phosphate atom to the second phosphate atom and when this chemical bond is broken, energy is released – and this is the energy we use. Below is a picture of the ATP molecule.

What Does ATP Look Like?

The ATP molecule essentially looks like the picture below:

Adenosine

High-energy phosphate bond. When broken, much energy is released.

Three phosphate atoms

As can be seen from the picture above, ATP is made of a molecule of adenosine (a type to sugar depicted on the right side of the picture) and three phosphate atoms (hanging off the side on the left of the picture). The short lines between the phosphate atoms represent chemical bonds that hold them together. There is energy contained within these bonds. As can be seen from the picture above, the chemical bond attached to the last phosphate is called a "high energy bond". This means that a large amount of energy is contained in this bond. When this chemical bond is broken, that energy is released. This is the energy that powers our activities.

How is ATP Made?

It should be understood that the human body has only a few seconds of ATP stored within it at any given time.[16]   Because of this, all activity would stop within a few seconds if ATP were not regenerated on a continual basis. ATP can be made over and over again via the following chemical pathways: the *ATP / CP system*, *glycolysis*, and the *Krebs cycle*.

- **The ATP/CP System.** The ATP/ CP system is an anaerobic energy pathway that consists of stored ATP and *creatine phosphate*. The few seconds of stored ATP, breaks down first to power our activity. During activities that require ATP to be regenerated at a faster rate than is normally possible by other means,

18

creatine phosphate is called into action. Creatine phosphate (CP) only comes into play during very short lasting, highly intense physical activities such as sprinting or lifting a very heavy weight. Acting like a supercharger for ATP production, creatine can help regenerate ATP for only a short period of time, approximately 30 seconds.[61] It's important to remember that the creatine energy system is not used during low intensity activities like walking, cycling or other activities that can be carried out for long periods of time. Likewise, creatine is not coming into play during relatively low intensity weight lifting programs like circuit training or programs where the resistance is lifted for 15 ore more repetitions. Further information about creatine can be found in the dietary supplements chapter. Some books may refer to the ATP/CP system as *phosphagens*. This name makes reference to the fact that both ATP and CP contain phosphate atoms.

More on ATP & CP

Some may be interested in the chemistry behind how ATP and CP work together. Below is a brief overview of how they work.

The removal of the high-energy phosphate from ATP yields a molecule called adenosine diphosphate (called ADP). The chemical reaction looks like this:

$$ATP \rightarrow ADP + P_i$$

P_i is the chemical symbol for an inorganic phosphate atom. Creatine phosphate can help reenergize ATP by donating its phosphate atom to ADP. The reaction looks like this:

$$CP + ADP \rightarrow ATP.$$

After being regenerated, ATP can once again breakdown, releasing its energy, so activity can continue.

- **Glycolysis.** Glycolysis refers to a series of chemical reactions in which ATP (energy) is made via the anaerobic (no oxygen needed) breakdown of carbohydrates. Glycolysis is also known as the *lactic acid system*, a name which refers to lactic acid, a metabolic byproduct formed during glycolysis. Lactic acid (also known as lactate) build-up inside muscles correlates with the burning sensation and fatigue that occurs when muscles are worked harder than they are used to.

The carbohydrate of choice used in glycolysis is the sugar, glucose (sometimes called *blood sugar*). When carbohydrates are eaten, they are chemically rearranged and transformed into the sugar glucose. Glucose, in turn, is stored in the body in the form of another molecule called *glycogen*. Remember, glycogen and glucose are basically the same thing. When glycogen is broken down, it releases glucose, which we can make energy out of.

What is Aerobic Glycolysis?

It should come as little surprise that the human body is far more complex than many suspect. The process of glycolysis highlights this fact very well. Glycolysis is usually considered an anaerobic energy-generating pathway. In other words, oxygen is not needed for glycolysis to occur. Under some circumstances however glycolysis can be aerobic and use oxygen. This process is sometimes called "aerobic glycolysis". During aerobic glycolysis, more ATP is made than during anaerobic glycolysis. The downside of this is that ATP is not made as fast.

Those struggling with which this concept and wondering which aspect of glycolysis—aerobic or anaerobic—occurs during different types of activities should remember that during higher intensity activity (when ATP must be made fast), anaerobic glycolysis predominates. During lower intensities of activity (when ATP doesn't need to be made as fast), aerobic glycolysis is more likely to occur.

- **The Krebs Cycle.** The Krebs cycle refers to a series of chemical reactions in which ATP is made from the breakdown of fat. The Krebs cycle is an aerobic pathway, meaning that it uses oxygen to metabolize fat. The Krebs cycle occurs in a specialized region of our cells called the *mitochondria*. It is within the mitochondria that the fat-brining enzymes are located. Two adaptations of aerobic exercise training that occur are that our mitochondria get bigger and we make more of them. Thus, as a result of aerobic exercise training, we are better able to use fat for fuel during exercise. In fact, aerobically trained individuals use more fat and less glycogen during submaximal exercise. Since the depletion of carbs (glycogen and glucose) can greatly hinder exercise performance, this means that exercise-trained muscles can workout longer because of their lower reliance on carbs and greater reliance on fat.

More on the Mitochondria

The mitochondria is often called "powerhouse of the cell". The reason for this is that fat is a very energy-dense molecule. Literally, hundreds of ATP molecules can be made from a single fat molecule. While indeed a powerhouse, another way to describe the mitochondria is to liken it to a battery. Those who have studied physics know that batteries, like those that power flashlights, CD players, cars etc. essentially work by separating positive and negative electrical charges. As these electrical charges come together, energy is produced. It turns out that the mitochondria also separates positive and negative electrical charges. As these electrical charges come together again, ATP is produced! So the mitochondria are essentially aerobic, rechargeable, fat-burning, batteries.

Another interesting fact about mitochondria is that when people regularly participate in aerobic exercise, the mitochondria of the cells of the body get bigger, and more numerous. Thus, a runner or cyclist would be expected to have more mitochondria in his/her cells than a sprinter or power lifter. The reason for this is that mitochondria are aerobic machines. When an aerobic stress is placed on the body on a regular basis (like working out several times a week), it sends a message to the cells to step up production of mitochondria to keep pace with the body's needs. The more mitochondria an athlete has, the better he/she is at burning fat.

The different energy systems described in this chapter have been listed separately to facilitate the learning process. However, it should be kept in mind that they are all used simultaneously, albeit to different degrees in the body. The intensity of the activity being performed and length of time (duration) that an activity is carried out, dictates whether a person is predominately making energy aerobically or anaerobically. If you are resting quietly while reading these words you are roughly 60% aerobic and 40% anaerobic. As intensity of activity increases, we start to make energy more anaerobically. Greater intensities of exercise mean a faster rate of energy production is needed, a task easily carried out by anaerobic energy production pathways like glycolysis and the ATP/CP system.

Chapter 3

Macronutrient Use During Exercise

Although previously mentioned, the fact that all macronutrients are always being used simultaneously deserves further discussion. All sources of calories — carbohydrate, fat and protein — are utilized or burned for fuel at the same time. However, the ratio or relative contribution of each nutrient varies with exercise intensity as well as with the duration at which exercise occurs. During activities that are of high intensity and short lasting (such as sprinting or heavy weight lifting), the body relies heavily upon the breakdown of immediately available ATP and the breakdown of carbohydrate. As the duration of the exercise increases, a gradual shift occurs where fat breakdown begins to contribute significantly to exercise energy demands. Thus, a continuum of macronutrient utilization exists where at one end (high intensity, short duration), ATP and carbohydrate breakdown contribute the abundance of energy needs, and at the other end of the continuum (low intensity, long duration), fat and carbohydrate use reign supreme. Another way of stating this is that at high intensity activity, *anaerobic* mechanisms of energy production predominate, whereas at lower intensity activities, *aerobic* metabolic processes prevail. This is why weight lifting is usually called anaerobic activity while walking and jogging are considered aerobic activities.

Exercise Intensity vs. Macronutrient Use	
Intensity/ Duration	**Fuels Used**
High Intensity, Short Lasting	ATP and Carbs
Low Intensity, Long Lasting	Carbs and Fats

Carbohydrate

Carbohydrates are the preferred fuel utilized during high intensity activity. As stated previously, the body relies more and more heavily upon carbohydrates as exercise intensity is increased. Glycogen, our storage form of carbohydrate, is concentrated within the muscles of the body as well as the liver. Glycogen stored within the muscles supplies large amounts of the energy in the transition from rest to moderate exercise as well as from moderate to intense exercise.[36] During moderate activity lasting at least 20 minutes, glycogen supplies between 40%-50% of the body's energy demands, with the other half being supplied by fat.[36] Only small amounts of protein are used during moderate exercise. If exercise were to continue in the absence of any nutrient replenishment, eventually glycogen levels would fall below that needed to maintain exercise, and fatigue would set in, hindering exercise performance.

Another area where carbohydrates might help during exercise is by boosting the immune system. It is well known that strenuous, long-duration aerobic exercise, like a marathon or triathlon can depress the immune system, resulting in a higher rate of colds developing in the days following the event. While not fully understood, research finds that carbohydrates consumed before and during prolonged high intensity aerobic exercise can support the immune system and as such may help reduce infections after an athletic event.[81]

Individuals should attempt to gain the bulk of their carbohydrates from complex carbohydrates such as fruits, vegetables and whole grains whenever possible. The reason for this is that complex carbohydrates are nutrient-dense foods. That is, they contain a lot of nutrients relative to their weight and tend not to raise blood sugar as fast as simple, relatively nutrient-deficient carbohydrates like candy, pies, cakes and soda.

Glycogen vs. Glucose

A key concept that is usually missed is that glucose and glycogen are essentially the same thing, just different forms of the same molecule. Glucose, a simple carbohydrate, is often called blood sugar. Many glucose molecules chemically linked together form the complex carbohydrate, glycogen. When glycogen breaks down, it releases individual glucose molecules, which cells can then use to make energy (ATP). The relationship between glucose and glycogen is analogous to that of water and ice. Both water and ice are the same thing. They just look different.

Fat

Fat represents the major fuel source used during light to moderate exercise. Fat released from the abdominal area represents a particularly active area of fat mobilization, compared to fat stores located in the hip and thigh areas[36]. Again, as exercise intensity increases, there is a shift from fat to carbohydrate for fuel. With exercise training, a number of positive changes occurs which facilitates the use of fat for fuel during exercise. These changes include.[36]:

- increased rate of release of fat from fat cells
- enhanced number of capillaries within trained muscles
- improved ability to transport fat through muscle cells
- improved ability to transport fat within muscle cells
- increased size and number of mitochondria
- enhanced quantity of fat-burning enzymes

Thus, exercise training (for example, three or more months of aerobic endurance training), produces favorable metabolic changes which facilitate the use of fat as a fuel source during exercise. Less fit individuals tend to rely more heavily on carbohydrates during exercise. This can result in the build up of lactic acid and is one of the reasons that unfit individuals may complain of muscle burning during exercise.

Fat Breakdown during Exercise

A common misconception is that one must exercise aerobically for at least 20 minutes before fat is broken down for energy. In actuality, fat breakdown begins to contribute to the body's energy needs after only a few minutes. However, it is only during longer durations of exercise that fat starts to contribute *significantly* to energy needs. For example, more fat is contributing to ATP needs after 20 minutes of exercise than after five minutes. Thus, large percentages of fat are used as a fuel source during exercise that is of *long duration and low intensity*. This makes perfect sense when one considers that it takes time to shuttle fat from the fat cells to the mitochondria and "chop" them up into smaller molecules to be burned for fuel.

There is an old saying that "fat burns in a carbohydrate flame". This refers to the fact that fat breakdown depends in part on metabolic byproducts of carbohydrate metabolism that help during the fat burning process. Reducing carbohydrates—as occurs through fasting or other low carbohydrate diets—reduces the amount of carbohydrate metabolic breakdown products available to assist in the fat burning process. This reduces fat breakdown and in the process, the body forms molecules called *ketones*. Ketones are acidic molecules which, in excess, alter the acidity of the body, thus hindering its proper functioning.

Fat breakdown is also hindered during long endurance exercise when carbo-hydrate intake is less than adequate. Runners and other endurance athletes sometimes refer to this depletion of carbohydrates during exercise as "hitting the wall".

The Skinny on the "Fat Burning" Program

Many people who have home exercise equipment or those who belong to health clubs have probably noticed that many of the treadmills, ellipticals and bikes have a "Fat Burn" program. This program is supposed to keep people in their "fat burning zone" and foster weight loss. Let's address this program for a moment and see what can be discovered.

The basis of the fat burning program is that we burn a greater percentage of fat at lower levels of exercise. In other words, we burn more fat at low intensity, long duration exercise. Let's take this reasoning and work backwards to its ultimate conclusion. Suppose a person is on a treadmill at 3 mph. Slowing the treadmill to 2 mph would burn more fat because it's a lower intensity. Slowing the treadmill to 1 mph would burn even more fat. Now stop exercising. Now sit down. Now go to sleep. Sleeping is actually the lowest intensity "activity" any of us can do and in fact studies show that about 70% of the calories burned during sleeping are coming from fat. The question then becomes, if sleeping burns the most fat, why can't people lose weight while sleeping? The answer is simple. We don't burn many calories sleeping. Calories burned—not fat burned—is the key to weight loss. We burn more calories exercising than sleeping.

The Fat Burn program does have its place because for an untrained person not used to exercise, it holds him/her to a relatively low intensity (usually around 60% of estimated max heart rate). At lower intensities, there is also a reduced risk of injury and in theory the person can do the activity for a longer period of time—which means more calories burned. Depending on the initial fitness level of the person, individuals may get used to the Fat Burn program after a few months. After that, they may want to opt for the "Cardio Program" that also is found on many treadmills etc. The Cardio Program holds people at a slightly higher level (about 80% of maximal heart rate).

Protein

As stated before, protein forms thousands of complex molecules in the body. Since protein is so crucial to health, it makes sense that it does not provide the bulk of the body's energy requirements at rest or during exercise. Compared to either carbohydrate or fat, protein contributes little to the energy requirements of exercise, with estimates of between 2 to 10 percent of total energy needs.[24] Thus, protein is not the fuel of choice during exercise. This is especially true in the individual who is supplied with adequate carbohydrate (thus, carbohydrate spares protein from being degraded in appreciable amounts during exercise). In those who have less than optimal carbohydrate and calorie intakes, protein is broken down in greater amounts.[45] In the long run, this may hinder muscle growth and thus, exercise performance.

Chapter 4

Nutrition and Exercise

This chapter will deal with the types and amounts of major nutrients that are thought to lead to optimal exercise capacity.

Carbohydrate

Exercise places a demand on the body that requires steady, relatively fast energy production. Because carbohydrates are relatively easy to make energy from, they represent the main macronutrient used by the body during exercise. This is especially true during activities that are of high intensity and short lasting such as resistance training. During exercise like cycling and running marathons, carbohydrates are often referred to as the "rate limiting nutrient". This phrase makes reference to the importance of carbohydrates to the continuation of exercise. In other words, when carbohydrate reserves are depleted, exercise stops, a process sometimes called "hitting the wall". Research finds that the human body has approximately 1200-1500 calories in the form of glycogen (the storage form of carbohydrates). This is enough energy to run non-stop for about 20 miles.[36] Because marathons, century bike rides, triathlons and other similar athletic events usually last longer than 20 miles, this is the reason that spectators will often see athletes eating during the events. If athletes didn't eat, they would eventually deplete their glycogen reserves, resulting in their dropping out of the race.

The importance of carbohydrates to exercise performance is the reason that they are often recommended in such high amounts for athletes. One of the functions of carbohydrates that often go unmentioned is that they help reduce protein breakdown. Thus, carbs help spare muscle protein (and other proteins) from being consumed for fuel.

In general, carbohydrates should contribute between 55-65% of total calorie intake. These carbohydrates should be derived from nutrient-dense complex carbohydrate foods such as fruits, vegetables and unprocessed grains. Again, complex carbs are stressed over simple carbs because of their higher nutrient content. Complex carbohydrates also tend not to cause the immediate spike in blood glucose levels that simple sugars do. In theory, a quick elevation in blood glucose levels could result in a rapid release of the hormone insulin, which tends to lower blood sugar and stimulate appetite. This, in turn, may cause lethargy and less than optimal performance during exercise.

Where Do the Extra Carbs Go?

As mentioned previously, roughly speaking, the body stores between 1200-1500 calories in the form of glycogen. Some readers may be wondering about the fate of carbs eaten after the body maxes out its storage ability? The answer is simple; the body converts the extra carbs to fat and stores them as fat. So, even though eating carbs is healthy, eating extra calories in the form carbohydrates can lead to greater weight gain in the form of fat.

The Glycemic Index

The glycemic index is an outgrowth of those dissatisfied with the classification of carbohydrates as merely simple and complex. Those dissenters maintained that judging carbs only by the number of sugars they contained did not adequately explain how those carbs functioned in the body. Out of this, the glycemic index was born.

The glycemic index (sometimes abbreviated GI) is a rating scale of how fast an ingested carbohydrate elevates blood sugar levels. The higher the number, the faster the carbohydrate will raise blood sugar. Glucose or white bread is usually used as a reference point and given a rating of 100, indicating that they raise blood sugar very fast. A food with a glycemic index of 70, for example, means that it will raise blood sugar levels 70% as great as the same amount of glucose or white bread would.[42]

Some have argued that eating foods with a low glycemic index is superior to eating foods with high glycemic index. For example, low glycemic index foods tend to make people feel fuller longer and might not stimulate appetite as much as foods with a high glycemic index. Some evidence suggests that a low glycemic index diet might also stave off type II diabetes and other diseases as well. However, determination of the glycemic index of a food can be difficult. For example, each of the following factors can affect the glycemic index of a food:[44]

- o Cooked vs. raw food
- o Fiber content of the food
- o Ripeness of the food (ripe banana vs. non-ripe for example)
- o Portion size (8 oz vs. 12 oz of a food for example)
- o Eating foods together gives a different GI than either food would alone

Foods with a rating of 70 or more are considered high glycemic index. Foods with a GI of 56 -69 are regarded as moderate glycemic index. Foods with a GI of less than 55 are usually thought of as low glycemic. Foods that contain no carbohydrates like meats do not have a glycemic index.

The Glycemic Index	
GI Range	**Meaning**
≥ 70	High GI
55-69	Medium GI
≤ 55	Low GI

Fruits and vegetables tend to be low glycemic index foods and, from a nutrition standpoint, they tend to offer more vitamins, minerals and fiber compared to higher index foods. Thus, fruits and vegetables figure prominently in glycemic index eating plans. The table below groups several different foods according to their glycemic index.

Glycemic Index of Foods		
Low GI (55 or less)	**Medium GI (55-69)**	**High GI (70 or above)**
• Milk	• Rye bread	• White bread
• Yoghurt	• Sodas	• French fries
• Banana	• Pineapple	• Corn Flakes™ cereal
• All Bran™ cereal	• Brown rice (steamed)	• Bran Flakes™ cereal
• Grapes	• White rice (Uncle Ben's, boiled)	• Cheerios™ cereal
• Pure Protein™ bar. Strawberry shortcake	• Met-Rx® meal replacement drink (Vanilla)	• Clif bar® Cookies and Cream
• Soy milk	• Pizza (cheese)	• Boiled potatoes
• Sweat Potatoes	• Oatmeal cookies	• Baked potatoes
• Nuts	• Ice cream (vanilla & chocolate)	• Jelly beans
• Baked Beans	• Angle food cake	• Coco Pops™ cereal

Adapted from glycemicindex.com

Glycemic Index & Exercise: Practical Uses

Currently, the role of glycemic index and its interaction with exercise performance remains controversial.[42,45] That being said, some practical uses of glycemic index can be utilized by athletes to help maximize their performance. Exercise, especially aerobic exercise, depletes glycogen levels. This lowering of glycogen is accompanied by an increase in an enzyme called glycogen synthase, which is responsible for making glycogen. Following exercise, humans have a window of opportunity of about 30-60 minutes when they are most capable of replenishing glycogen reserves. This is why it is often recommended that athletes eat as soon as possible after exercise. If this tactic of eating 30-60 minutes after exercise were to be combined with eating a high glycemic index food, the result might equal even greater glycogen storage.[69] This, in turn, might benefit athletes involved in daily bouts of long-duration exercise like the Tour de France, the Olympics or other similarly grueling athletic events. For those involved in strength training, eating some protein along with a high glycemic index food might, in theory, enhance the uptake of amino acids, needed to help rebuild muscle.

During long duration exercise, like running a marathon, athletes traditionally eat carbohydrates to maintain blood sugar levels and prevent glycogen depletion. The consumption of high glycemic index foods during this time might decrease exercise performance by causing large spikes in insulin which might lower blood sugar too much. In contrast, low to moderate glycemic index foods, which do not dramatically increase insulin, may be a better choice during exercise. This is the reason that spectators of marathons, triathlons and other such events may often see athletes eating bananas during the event. Bananas are a classic low glycemic index food.

Glycemic Index and Weight Loss?

Some have argued that eating foods according to their glycemic index can promote optimal weight loss. According the American Dietetic Association however there is not enough evidence to warrant this conclusion.[70] Low glycemic index foods tend to include many fruits and vegetables which are usually recommended to those looking to shed excess weight. Most evidence to date finds that it is the reduced calories associated with eating these foods as opposed to their GI that is most important for weight loss.

The Glycemic Load

The concept of glycemic load is an extension of glycemic index. Remember that the glycemic index can be affected by the amount of food eaten. This makes a glycemic index diet rather difficult to follow. The glycemic load (sometimes abbreviated as "GL") may, according to some, be a better way to eat.

The glycemic load is defined as the glycemic index of a food multiplied by the number of grams of carbohydrate eaten. The resulting number is then divided by 100.[71] Some research finds that people who eat a high glycemic load diet suffer from more diseases like diabetes.[71] Higher glycemic load diets might also be linked to elevated CRP levels.[71] C reactive protein (CRP) is a compound which is implicated in the development of heart disease. Foods such as fruits and vegetables, grains and beans tend to have a low glycemic load. These foods also tend to have a low glycemic index as well.

Foods with a GL of 10 or less are called low glycemic load foods. Those with a GL of 10-19 are medium glycemic index foods. Foods with a GL or more than 20 are considered high glycemic load foods.

The Glycemic Load	
GL Range	**Meaning**
≤ 10	Low GL
11 to 19	Medium GL
≥ 20	High GL

Glycemic Index & Glycemic Load of Selected Foods			
Food	**Amount**	**Glycemic Index**	**Glycemic Load**
Baked potatoes	1 medium	85	26
Jelly beans	1 oz	78	22
White rice	1 cup	64	23
Brown rice	1 cup	55	18
Orange	1 medium	42	5
All Bran™ cereal	1 cup	38	9
Cornflakes	1 cup	81	21
Skim milk	1 cup	32	4

Deciphering glycemic index and glycemic load can be a challenge. The table below shows how the ranking scales of each compare.

Glycemic Index vs. Glycemic Load: How they Compare		
	GI Range	**GL Range**
Low	< 55	<10
Medium	55 to 69	11 to 19
High	≥ 70	≥ 20

The evidence linking low glycemic index and low glycemic load diets to reduced disease risk is interesting. Those who are confused as to which is best should remember that both viewpoints emphasize the value of complex carbohydrates, fruits, vegetables, grains and beans. This is, for the most part, still in line with popular dietary recommendations such as those advocated by the American Dietetic Association. Thus, people eating healthy diets consisting of grains, vegetables, fruits and legumes may already be adhering to recommendations advocated by low glycemic index and low glycemic load philosophies. Remembering this fact may save people time and energy as they further investigate this topic.

Protein

Most of the energy used during exercise comes from carbs and fats. Protein contributes little energy during exercise. The Recommended Dietary Allowance (RDA) for protein for *non-exercising* individuals is 0.8 grams per kilogram of body weight (kg/BW).[134] In real life terms, this also equals 0.36 grams per pound. Thus, protein intake depends in part on how much a person weighs. For example, a person weighing 150 lbs (68 kg) will have a protein RDA of 68 kg X 0.8 = 55.5 grams (about two ounces) of protein. A person who weighs 200 lbs will have an RDA of about 73 grams of protein. While studies find that the recommendation of 0.8 grams/kilogram is enough for most active individuals[36], other recommendations call for somewhat higher amounts of protein for those who exercise regularly or intensely.[30,134]

Estimated Protein Requirements for Exercise	
Goal	Amount
Maintaining Muscle	1.2 - 1.3 g/Kg/BW
Building Muscle	1.4 - 1.8 g/Kg/BW

Note: 1 kilogram = 2.2 pounds. BW = body weight. The lower amounts are also appropriate for those involved in endurance athletic events

The protein requirements in the table above are not engraved in stone and are offered as a guideline when fitness professionals are asked about how much protein a strength trainer should consume. Because people differ in their fitness levels, nutrition habits and exercise programs, it is possible that for some individuals, muscle mass and strength may actually increase by use of the "maintaining muscle" recommendations.

It is often stated by nutrition professionals that the average non-exercising American often exceeds the RDA for protein.[36] Some research has noted that US men age 20 and over consume 152% of the RDA for protein while women consume 127%.[78] As stated previously, protein is not the fuel of choice during exercise. Thus, it is usually not used in large quantities during athletic events. Rather, carbohydrate and fat contribute greater amounts of energy during periods of physical activity. That being said the "optimal" amount of protein necessary for "optimal" exercise performance is not currently known. Research suggests however that for most people, it is probably within the 1.2-1.8 g/kg BW range cited previously.[134]

The branched-chain amino acids (leucine, isoleucine and valine) are used for fuel during exercise and are sometimes supplemented by those looking to improve exercise capacity. Some research hints that the branch chain amino acids limit the entry of the amino acid, tryptophan into the brain. Given that tryptophan helps make the neuro-chemical, serotonin, which plays a role in sleep, adding BCAAs to the diet might lower serotonin levels and thus extend the time before fatigue sets in. This is an intriguing theory, and also a controversial one; studies to date have been unable to show conclusively that ingestion of branched-chain amino acids during exercise enhances athletic performance.[32] If BCAAs work, they might best suited for professional athletes and those who take part in endurance events like marathons and long range cycling events.

When people discuss protein they often wonder when is the best time to eat it – before or after exercise. In other words, which leads to greater muscle growth? Currently much evidence supports the notion that eating protein immediately (i.e. within 1 hour) after exercise is superior to eating it prior to exercise.[134] In addition, combining protein with carbohydrate is better still given that carbs stimulate insulin which helps with the assimilation of amino acids.

Another question that often comes up with respect to protein is how much can be absorbed in a meal? Many people reading these words have probably heard that people can only absorb 35-40 grams of protein per meal. In reality there is no proof of this. Protein is highly absorbed by the body with most of what you eat being absorbed. While flawed, the statement can be said to have some merit because it helps people remember that carbs (and even fats) are important to a healthy diet.

High Protein Diets & Weight Loss

Some people attempting to lose weight opt to increase the amount of protein in their diet. This is either accomplished by consuming more protein-containing foods or high-protein shakes, food bars or other supplements. Protein may be effective in this regard for a few reasons. First. Protein is relatively low in calories, containing roughly 4 calories per gram. Eating protein at the expense of other higher calorie foods like fats can create a calorie deficit which could foster weight loss. Second, protein tends to make people feel fuller longer than carbohydrates. Thus, people who eat protein may not feel hungry as often which also might promote a reduced level of calories consumed. Third, protein has a mild thermogenic effect. The thermic effect of food (sometimes abbreviated as TEF) relates to how much energy the body must invest to metabolize (digest, process, transport, etc.) the food in question. Some estimates put the thermic effect of protein to be almost 30% greater than fat (which has the lowest TEF and is thus the most easily assimilated macronutrient). So, higher protein diets, might slightly and temporarily elevate metabolism (the speed we burn calories) which in turn might result in more calories being burned over time. Forth, protein promotes the loss of water from the body. When protein is metabolized it makes a compound called urea, which is flushed from the body in the urine. Water is used in the process. This dehydration aspect of protein is sometimes used by bodybuilders to give them a more vascular appearance.

How Protein Might Help Weight Loss
1. Protein is low in calories
2. Protein slows digestion
3. Protein boosts metabolism
4. Protein promotes water loss

While protein can play a beneficial role in helping people lose weight, protein alone at the expense of other healthy foods is not a sensible road to weight loss. What is most effective for weight reduction is reducing the number of calories eaten. One drawback to higher protein diets is that they are not the best for people who exercise regularly. Because the body relies on carbohydrates and fat to power most activities, increasing protein consumption may leave some with reduced energy levels which could hinder athletic performance. Thus, people on high protein diets (at the expense of carbs and/or fat) should expect that their athletic performance, as well as their staying ability in the gym, may decrease.

Are Protein Supplements Needed?

It is often said that all the protein needed to help build muscle can easily be obtained from a healthy diet. This is in fact true, however, some people may find it easier to add a protein bar or protein shake to their diet as added insurance to help make up for what they think they may be missing. A wide array of protein supplements are available and more are created all the time to accommodate the needs of consumers. Like all supplements, protein bars, shakes and other products are designed to *supplement* the diet and not take the place of food. Research does exist showing that protein supplements can indeed contribute to muscle growth and quality made supplements are expected to be as good as protein-containing food for this purpose.

The big advantage of protein supplements, however, is their convenience. While this can be an asset to those with busy schedules, quality protein supplements may also benefit those who have trouble eating, like seniors. Seniors usually don't eat as much as they should and may have trouble chewing because of dentures. Lack of adequate dietary protein could result in the body cannibalizing its own protein reserves, like those found in muscle. In this instance, the addition of a quality protein supplement to their diet may help seniors preserve lean muscle mass. The safeguarding of muscle mass as one grows older can have a profound influence on the quality (and quantity) of life by helping keep muscles strong and offsetting sarcopenia (age-related muscle loss). Additional protein might also have other benefits such as helping maintain strong immune systems and other vital functions as well. When discussing protein with those with special needs such as seniors, the fitness professional should remember that while a crucial nutrient, too much protein might influence bone loss, something that seniors can do without.

Ultimately the decision to use a protein supplement is an individual one. Before deciding on a protein supplement the fitness professional should first determine how much protein (and calories) are currently being consumed by the individual. This can sometimes be determined by having the client fill out a 3 day food journal. After this is known, the fitness professional can weigh this information against factors such as the frequency and intensity of exercise being performed as well as the client's goals and whether or not those goals are being achieved. Remember, not all protein supplements may be appropriate for everyone. Calorie and protein content as well as that of fat and other nutrients can vary greatly from product to product. The following tables are a brief list of some commercially available protein supplements with a breakdown of their more popular nutrients.

Protein Drinks

Product	Calories	Protein (g)	Total Fat (g)	Total Carbs (g)	Sugars (g)
ABB Super High Protein Formula Extreme Body RTD 50. Milk Chocolate. (12 can =11 oz)	250	50	1.5	8	4
GNC Pro Performance 50 Grand Slam™ Milk Chocolate. (1 can=15 oz)	270	50	2	12	4
EAS Myoplex Carb Sense Rich Dark Chocolate. (1carton= 11oz)	140	25	4	5	<1

Protein Powders

Product	Calories	Protein (g)	Total Fat (g)	Total Carbs (g)	Sugars (g)
Accelerade® All Natural Protein, Orange (1 scoop=31 g) Accelerade.com	120	5	1	1	20
Designer Whey Protein. Strawberry (1 scoop, ~24g). Designerwhey.com	90	18	1.0	2	2
Kashi Go Lean® Chocolate (2 scoops = 60g). kashi.com	220	22	1	31	22

Protein Bars

Product	Calories	Protein (g)	Total Fat (g)	Total Carbs (g)	Sugars (g)
Balance® Cookie Dough (1 bar=50g). Balance.com	200	15	6	22	18
MET-Rx® Big 100 Chocolate Chip Cookie Dough (1bar=100g) Metrx.com	360	27	5	51	26
Powerbar® Cookies & Cream (1bar=65 g) Powerbar.com	240	9	3.5	45	20

Can We Eat Too Much Protein?

A common question that often arises when discussing protein is whether it is possible to consume too much? The short answer to this is yes; of course it is, especially if protein is used at the expense of other nutritious foods. Most people however are looking for a specific amount of protein, past which side effects might start to show up. The answer to this question might be particularly important in people who are using high protein diet supplements. Most experts stipulate that no more than 2 grams of protein per kilogram of body weight be consumed. The often cited reasons for this are mostly to do with protein over-stressing kidneys and causing kidney problems. One review of the literature concerning this issue however, found that high protein diets (defined as 1.5 grams per kilogram of body weight) do not appear harmful to the kidneys of healthy adults.[72] More research needs to be conducted to verify these conclusions and whether or not high protein diets (in excess of 1.5 grams per kilogram of body weight) are detrimental to kidney function in healthy adults. Many professional athletes commonly use more than 2 grams of protein per kilogram of body weight. From this, some might contend that high protein diets are less risky than thought. Professional athletes do tend to be in better shape than most individuals, which might make extrapolating this to the general public difficult. Also, high protein intakes would not be appropriate for those who have liver or kidney problems or other medical disorders.

Another often cited potential side effect of high protein diets concerns its effect on bones. Specifically, protein is known to leach calcium from the bones. This has caused some to speculate that high protein diets may be a risk factor for osteoporosis. Research however does not universally support this theory.[134] When examining this it is interesting to look at those who eat the most protein. Specifically, athletes like bodybuilders and powerlifters traditionally eat large amounts of protein, usually far in excess of the RDA. Yet osteoporosis is not a problem for these individuals. Is it possible that any deleterious effects of protein on bones might be offset by the positive effects of resistance training? It's an interesting theory and one worthy of further study.

Protein and Vegetarians

Some people choose to consume a diet that is composed of only fruits and vegetables. The fitness professional should have a grasp of the nuances of vegetarianism and its role in exercise and exercise performance. People have a variety of motives behind their choice to become a vegetarian, including religious, health and ethical reasons to name a few. Research finds that being a vegetarian does have some health benefits such as less risk of a variety of diseases. Within the lifestyle of vegetarianism, several subgroups exist:[12]

- **Lacto-ovo-vegetarians**: eat vegetables, milk and eggs but not meat or seafood.

- **Lacto-vegetarian:** consume vegetables, milk and milk products but not eggs.

- **Ovo-vegetarians**: consume vegetables and eggs but not milk or milk products.

- *Fruitarians*: consume only fruits and nuts.

As stated in previous sections, some amino acids are essential and must be obtained from the diet (or through supplements). Foods such as meat, fish and poultry that contain all of the essential amino acids in the right amounts are often called *complete* proteins. The compliment of essential amino acids in vegetables tend to be less than that of meats and as such, vegetables are usually referred to as *incomplete proteins*. However the decision to become a vegetarian does not preclude one from building muscle or competing athletically. While many foods the vegetarian may consume are by themselves *incomplete* proteins, when combined with other foods, they together can unite to make a complete protein source. For example, the following foods, when combined together will result in a complete, high quality, protein, and can help build muscle:[30]

- Rice and beans
- Corn and beans
- Corn and lima beans
- Pasta and bean soup

Another important thing to remember is that the above foods do not have to be eaten at the same meal to be effective. Consuming complementary incomplete proteins within 24 hours of each other is just as effective as if they were eaten at the same time.[12] Thus, eating meat does not preclude one from staying healthy and building muscle. In fact, on some levels, vegetarians are more healthy than those whose diet consists of beef and other meat products in that they tend to develop less obesity, cancer, diabetes and heart disease than meat eaters.

Another option for vegetarians is to eat soy. While derived from plants, soy is a complete protein and as such is also a viable alternative for those who do not consume meat. Studies show that diets containing 25-50 grams of soy a day can also help lower cholesterol levels.

One possible drawback to a strict non-animal containing diet is that vegetarians may be deficient in some vitamins and minerals—specifically, vitamin B_{12}, iron and zinc.[30] These deficiencies however can be easily dealt with by the use of a daily multivitamin containing the RDA for all the vitamins and minerals.

Fat

Contrary to what some may have been told, fat is not a useless macronutrient. Fat provides an abundance of the body's energy needs during exercise. Examples of activities that may use fat as a fuel source include walking, swimming, biking, hiking and bicycling. Comparatively, little fat is utilized for fuel during resistance training programs. While in the past, the news media has portrayed fat as an undesirable nutrient, the fitness professional should recognize that fat is a valuable asset to those who are involved in exercise training. Because fat is an energy-dense nutrient (i.e., it contains 9 calories per gram), it is much easier to add extra needed calories to the diet using fat—compared to protein or carbohydrate—in order to maintain body weight and muscle mass. In addition, some evidence finds that the normal rise in testosterone that occurs following resistance training is *decreased* in those who consume a low fat diet.[58]

Fat basically comes in three different forms: *monounsaturated* fat, *polyunsaturated* fat and *saturated* fat. From a health standpoint the mono and polyunsaturated fats tend to better for us. Diets high in saturated fats have been shown to raise the risk of heart disease. From a calorie standpoint however, all types of fat have 9 calories per gram. This is important to remember because it is possible to gain weight even if using a diet that's high in healthy fats. Remember, calories are the key to weight loss (and weight gain)—not fat.

Current recommendations for this macronutrient advocate that no more than 30% of total daily calorie intake should be derived from fats, with the majority of this amount coming from unsaturated fats. Some diets may advocate lower amounts of fat however fat makes food taste good and helps maintain the feeling of "fullness" longer. Thus, diets lower than 30% fat may be more difficult to maintain for the long haul.

High Fat Diets and Exercise Performance

Since fat provides a wealth of energy during exercise, some may wonder if eating a high fat can boost exercise performance? The answer to this questions appears to be no. When athletes are placed on diets containing various amounts of fat, higher fat diets have not shown to improve exercise performance.[69]

Trans Fats

As saturated fats started to fall out of favor with the public, some companies began using partially hydrogenated fats instead. Partially hydrogenated fats are less saturated than saturated fats and were at one time thought to be a more healthier alternative. Research shows that during the process of making partially hydrogenated fats, trans fats are created. Because of this, trans fatty acids are sometimes found in products that contain saturated fats like baked goods and fast foods. Trans fats are on the radar screens of a lot of nutritionists because they appear to decrease HDL and increase LDL By lowering HDL and increasing LDL, trans fats have the potential to clog arteries and elevate heart disease risk. Because of this, the FDA now mandates that food labels list trans fats. Foods that have less than 0.5 grams of trans fats per serving can say they have zero trans fats. However "per serving" is the important part. For example, if a trans fat free food has 10 servings and all of it is eaten, in theory you may have eaten 0.5 x 10 = 5grams of trans fats.

Chapter 5

Boosting Exercise Performance

Athletes, both professional and weekend warrior are forever trying different ways to both improve their exercise performance and accelerate the how fast they adapt to exercise. This chapter reviews some of the more popular methods used by people and provides a working understanding of those which might help and those which might be less effective.

Carbohydrate Loading

This method of boosting exercise performance has been used by triathletes and other ulta-endurance athletes for years. Technically called *glycogen super-compensation*, carbohydrate loading (or simply "carbo loading"), takes advantage of our enhanced ability to store carbohydrate (glycogen) after a period of carbohydrate restriction. The action of cutting back on carbs causes the body to increase its output of an enzyme called glycogen synthase. Glycogen synthase helps make glycogen. Thus, an increase in this enzyme might help us load up on glycogen when we eat carbs again.

While a number of *recipes* to achieve this glycogen loading effect exist, typically an athlete will participate in aerobic exercise for approximately 7-10 days before a competition to purposely exhaust his/her glycogen reserves. This is accompanied by a conscious decision to restrict the consumption of carbohydrates (sometimes only 100 g of carbs per day are eaten! This is very low and people should expect that their ability to exercise will drastically decrease during this time). At approximately three to four days before the event, people then eat a high-carbohydrate diet (upwards of 400 – 700 grams of carbs per day). Research finds that carbo-loading might lead to a 50%-100% increase in the amount of glycogen stored. For those who don't wish to do any math, another version calls for simply increasing carbohydrate intake while cutting back on the volume of exercise performed.

Studies show that carbo-loading seems to work best for aerobic endurance events lasting more than 90 minutes.[36] It would be expected to be less effective for those who take part in 5K runs or who workout a few days a week at the gym. Whether or not carbo-loading improves exercise performance for those who strength train needs more study.[30]

A word of caution for those considering carbo-loading: The body will eventually get used to it, making it less effective. Thus, this technique is not something to do on a regular basis. In addition, it is probably wise to experiment with carbo-loading before the actual athletic event. This way, people can see how they react to it.

Caffeine Supplementation

Caffeine, a stimulant found in coffee, caffeinated sodas and other commercially available products is often used by athletes to boost mental alertness, improve reaction time and enhance overall exercise performance. Studies show that caffeine can:

1. promote the release of adrenaline (epinephrine), a stimulating hormone, from the adrenal glands
2. stimulate the release of calcium from cells which in turn helps muscle contraction
3. prompt the release of fatty acids into the blood where they can be burned for fuel
4. heighten overall psychological and physiological arousal which can help improve reaction time and exercise performance

Most of the evidence for caffeine's improvement of exercise performance involves long duration aerobic events like marathons. The evidence for caffeine's effects on improving short, high intensity events like sprinting are mixed with some finding it may help and other studies hinting it doesn't. Studies of caffeine and exercise have used between 2-10 mg/ kg. The effect of caffeine probably varies from person to person and habitual use of caffeine may impact how effective it is. It should be noted that while commonly used by millions of people around the world, caffeine is not with out risks. Doses of over 200 mg a day may speed heart rate and interfere with sleeping. Doses above 10 grams of caffeine a day (150 mg/kg) can be fatal. Competitive athletes should remember that high doses of caffeine are also illegal in the Olympics.

Water

As important as protein, fat, carbohydrate, vitamins and minerals are to the maintenance of health and exercise performance, water is equally as important. Few things drive this fact home better than when one considers that the average person can usually last for months without food, yet will die after about a week without water. Based on this, water could even be considered the most important nutrient of all. Depending on age, gender and body composition, water makes up between 40%-70% of the mass of the body.[36] With respect to muscle and fat, water comprises 65-75% and 50% respectively.[36]

Functions of Water

Water serves a variety of purposes in the body. For example:

- Water helps transport nutrients and gasses throughout the body.
- Water serves as a medium for a vast array of chemical reactions.
- Water helps lubricate joints.

- Water helps dissipate excess heat, thus helping maintain a constant body temperature.

Consequences of Dehydration

Dehydration refers to a situation when fluid intake does not match fluid loss.[36] Almost all physical exertion results in some fluid loss. For example, a moderate one hour exercise session can result in a loss of between 0.5 to 1.5 liters of sweat.[36] Higher intensity exercise, especially in a hot environment, increases fluid loss even more. Studies show that a fluid loss of only two percent of body weight can significantly decrease exercise performance.[21]

The average person consumes approximately 91 ounces of water each day.[36] Since fluid loss via perspiration can increase dramatically during times of physical activity, fluid intake may increase to six times over normal levels during these periods. During exercise in high heat and humidity, fluid loss may exceed ten pounds.[32]

How Water is Lost From the Body

There are essentially four ways water is lost from the body:

1. Water loss through the skin. This form of water loss occurs when water is lost from the sweat glands of the body and serves as a way in which the body cools itself. The body is constantly cooling itself via this mechanism. This small amount of constant sweat is called *insensible perspiration*.

2. Water loss as water vapor. This represents water that is lost when we exhale.

3. Water loss from urine. The average loss of water from urine is approximately 1.5 quarts per day.

4. Water loss in feces. While this may not be immediately considered, fluid is lost in the feces. In fact, water makes up about 70% of fecal matter.[36] The loss of fluid though the feces can increase dramatically during periods of diarrhea.

Fluid Intake and Exercise

Prior to exercise, individuals should be well hydrated. Thus, fluid intake should start before exercise even begins. This is especially try for cyclists, triathletes and other similar athletes. A quick way to check for ample hydration is to observe the color of urine. Urine that is dark and which has a strong odor may be an indicator of less than adequate hydration.[36] Fluid hydration recommendations call for drinking approximately 17-20 ounces two to three hours before exercise and approximately seven to ten ounces of fluid ten to 20 minutes before exercise.[15] This should allow ample time for the passage of fluid into the body. During exercise, individuals should consume seven to ten ounces every ten to 20 minutes for the duration of the event. Following exercise, it is not uncommon to lose weight via fluid loss from sweat. To determine if weight loss has occurred following exercise, individuals should weigh themselves before and after physical activity. New recommendations on fluid replacement following exercise call for the ingestion of three cups (24 ounces) of fluid for every pound of fluid lost during exercise.[15] Ideally, this fluid should be consumed within two hours following exercise.[15] Properly scheduling fluid replacement before, during and after exercise will help ensure that circulation and sweating each work at optimum levels.

| Fluids: Before, During and After Exercise ||
Time	Fluid Intake
• 10-20 before exercise	7-10 oz
• During exercise	7-10 oz every 10-20 min
• After exercise	24 oz per pound lost

Alcohol

Alcohol is a poor substitute for water during athletics because it dehydrates the body and impairs exercise performance. Alcohol is a depressant to the nervous system which further reduces athletic performance by decreasing balance and coordination. Because alcohol is a diuretic, it speeds the loss of water, vitamins and minerals including thiamin, vitamin B_6 and calcium.[30] In addition to being devoid of any significant vitamins, minerals or other nutrients, alcohol is also a potent source of calories. Every gram of alcohol contains 7 calories. That is almost as much as is contained in fat (9 calories/ gram). While evidence does exist showing that moderate alcohol consumption may elevate HDL levels, so, too, does exercise. Excessive alcohol consumption can raise blood pressure and elevate triglyceride levels.[30] It might also reduce glycogen re-storage and testosterone production.

Sports Drinks

Some may opt to drink beverages other than water such as "sports drinks". Consuming these drinks may actually have a benefit by enhancing fluid consumption because they taste good. One study examined the level of voluntary fluid intake between plain water, grape-flavored water or grape-flavored water containing 6 percent carbohydrate and salts, as electrolytes.[35] This study found that the beverage containing the carbohydrates and salts resulted in the most volume of fluid ingested.

Another advantage of sports drinks occurs during exercise that lasts longer than 1 to 2 hours, especially in the heat. The carbohydrates contained in sports drinks help reduce the utilization of muscle glycogen. This in turn can help improve exercise performance. It's important to note that not all sport drinks are alike. Some in fact may just be fancy sugar water. When choosing sports drinks, look for those which contain less than 8% carbohydrate.[30] Beverages containing high doses of simple sugars may slow the absorption of the fluid, which in turn may decrease exercise performance. The type of carbohydrate used in sports drinks may also be a factor to consider. For example, high levels of the sugar, fructose, in drinks may promote slower absorption than drinks containing other sugars like glucose.

Glutamine

Glutamine is an amino acid—one of the building blocks that make up protein. Glutamine is usually labeled a *non-essential* amino acid, because we have the ability to make it as needed. However, it appears that our need for glutamine may increase during certain conditions, like surgery or chronic, debilitating disease. It is for this reason that glutamine is sometimes called a *conditionally* essential amino acid. Research finds that when glutamine is given intravenously to sick people that it can help improve body weight and muscle mass and reduce the time one spends in the hospital.[74] Some wonder if this same effect might also be had by healthy people who exercise. Research to date of healthy people who exercise has not observed that glutamine improves strength or athletic performance.[75] Many athletes like bodybuilders however use glutamine not to make them stronger but rather to slow muscle breakdown and speed up the time it takes them to recover following repeated bouts of high intensity exercise. In theory, this might be possible but good scientific support for glutamine helping in this regard is lacking. Some research has noted that orally-taken glutamine, when used in conjunction with the amino acid arginine and a supplement called HMB may hold promise in reducing muscle loss in those with cancer and HIV.[76] Whether or not these same results would be obtained by healthy people, like bodybuilders is less well known. For additional and expanded information on glutamine and well over 100 other popular supplements, read my book, *Nutritional Supplements: What Works and Why* available at www.Joe-Cannon.com.

Blood Doping

Blood doping is a dangerous practice often used by some elite cyclists and marathoners and involves donating and storing one's own blood. The blood is then pumped back into the athlete's body before the race. This is done to boost the concentration of oxygen carrying red blood cells. More red blood cells mean greater oxygen carrying capacity which in turn might mean improved ability to exercise longer and at a higher intensity. One of the problems with blood doping is that when athletes exercise, they tend to sweat. This loss of fluid from the body means the blood gets thicker. This in turn, puts an added stress on the heart as it works harder to pump the thicker blood. Heart attacks and death have been known to occur following blood doping and for this reason it is illegal in many sports.

Another strategy sometimes employed is to use a drug called EPO. EPO is a synthetic version of erythropoietin, a hormone that makes red blood cells. Thus, by using EPO, red blood cell production is increased. This too, can result in increased blood viscosity which in turn can be hazardous to health for the same reasons mentioned previously. The use of EPO is also illegal in most sports.

Training at Higher Altitudes

When preparing for a race or other athletic event, some athletes, train at locations that are at higher altitudes than where the event will take place. Higher altitudes generally mean less oxygen is available for the person to breath. The body then adapts to this lack of oxygen by naturally making more red blood cells (erythrocytes). When the athlete returns to lower elevations, he/she may have more stamina and improved exercise performance because of their greater oxygen carrying capacity. Keep in mind that increases in red blood cell levels do not occur overnight. Rather, several weeks of living and exercising at higher altitudes may be needed before significant changes are observed. Another consideration when training at higher altitudes involves the increased use of protein for fuel that might occur as a result of the body burning more calories than it normally does at lower elevations. This could result in muscle loss and reduced exercise performance. Increased calorie needs might also be expected if the athlete is training at a higher altitude that is also cold. These caveats not withstanding, training at higher altitudes has been called "natural blood doping" by some because of its ability to boost performance. Training at higher altitudes however is not an illegal practice, unlike *real* blood doping which is.

Vitamin B-12 Supplements

Vitamin B-12 is needed for the production of red blood cells, which carry oxygen. Thus, like other practices described above, the rationale behind using vitamin B-12 supplements is that the nutrient might boost red blood cell production, which in turn, might improve exercise performance. To date however research has not noted improvements in exercise ability following vitamin B-12 supplementation in healthy people. It is noteworthy to mention that unlike many of the B vitamins which are excreted regularly, vitamin B-12 is stored for many years in the body. Thus, deficiencies in this vitamin are unlikely, especially in athletes and regular exercisers who are not vegetarians and likely eating a healthy diet or using supplements which contain this nutrient.

Iron Supplements

The mineral iron is crucial for red blood cells to carry oxygen. As such, some people may use iron supplements in the hopes that it will help their blood transport more oxygen, battle exercise fatigue and improve overall exercise capacity. For those who have been diagnosed with iron-deficiency anemia, iron supplements may in fact be helpful and improve exercise performance. For those who are not anemic however, iron supplements do not appear to be of benefit. When used in excess, iron can be dangerous especially for those who have a rare genetic condition called hemochromotosis (iron overload disease). In this disorder iron absorption is enhanced and can lead to a wide spectrum of problems ranging from joint pain and fatigue to liver disorders and even death. Iron is also a controversial mineral for men where some research links it as a possible contributor to heart disease. This is the reason that many "men's formula" multi-vitamins do not contain iron. Iron is found in meats as well as many green vegetables and legumes. Unless prescribed by a doctor, iron supplements cannot be recommended.

Sodium Bicarbonate

The letters pH refer to a zero to 14 scale that is often used in chemistry to measure acidity levels. Lower pH numbers indicate greater acidity and higher numbers reflect alkalinity. Acids, such as lactic acid created during exercise can decrease exercise performance by inducing fatigue and reducing the power capacity of muscles. Given this fact, some athletes may attempt to help the body better buffer against increases in acid production in the hopes of extending the time before fatigue sets in. Normally this practice involves the use of baking soda (sodium bicarbonate) before an athletic event. Research, while mixed, does hint that sodium bicarbonate may be of help to athletes involved not only in highly anaerobic types of activity like sprinting but also might benefit those who take part in marathons and triathlons. Normally bicarbonate is used one to two hours before a competition at a concentration of about 300 milligrams per kilogram of body weight.[79] Some research suggests this practice may help shave a few seconds off an athlete's speed, which in competitive events, is significant. Those considering sodium bicarbonate should experiment with it before their actual athlete event to see how their body's respond. Studies indicate that sodium bicarbonate may cause diarrhea and abdominal pain one to two hours after ingestion.

Chapter 6

Vitamins & Minerals

Vitamins

Vitamins are organic compounds needed in small amounts to ensure health. The term *organic* is a reference to the fact that vitamins contain the element carbon which is fundamental to all life on earth. To be classified as a vitamin, the substance in question must either:

1. not naturally be made in the body

2. be associated with a disease or condition, if the substance is missing from the diet

The classic example often used to describe vitamins is the story of vitamin C where hundreds of years ago, British sailors on long sea voyages would develop scurvy, a condition that if not corrected is fatal. In time it was discovered that eating citrus fruits prevented scurvy from occurring. This lead to the widespread use of limes and other citrus fruits by sailors in the British Navy. Ultimately, the compound in citrus fruits that prevented scurvy was found to be vitamin C. It is from the use of limes by British sailors that they earned the popular nickname, *limeys*.

As mentioned above, the body generally cannot make vitamins. Thus, vitamins must either be obtained from food or from the use of supplements. The exception to this rule is vitamin D which can be made upon exposure to sunlight. Vitamins can be classified according to whether they dissolve in fat or water. The fat-soluble vitamins are vitamins A, E, D and vitamin K. The water-soluble vitamins are vitamin C and the B complex family of vitamins.

The Fat-Soluble Vitamins

Vitamins A, E, D and K are the fat-soluble vitamins. They are called fat soluble because they are best absorbed when consumed with some fat. This is one of the reasons that it is sometimes recommended that multivitamins be taken with meals.

The fat soluble vitamins serve an array of purposes. For example, vitamin A aids with the proper functioning of the eyes.[36] Vitamin E helps blood circulate more freely by helping reduce the likelihood of blood clotting inside the body. Vitamin K helps the blood to clot when we have been cut or injured. Lastly, one of the functions of vitamin D is that it helps with proper bone development.

Because the human body is able to store fat-soluble vitamins for great lengths of time (years in some cases), they do not need to be ingested daily.[36] In addition, ingesting fat-soluble vitamins in excess of their recommended dietary allowance is usually cautioned against by medical professionals because of the possibility of toxic reactions. For example, pregnant women who consume large amounts of vitamin A early in their pregnancy have an increased risk of birth defects.[36] In children, high intakes of vitamin A can result in itchy skin as well as swelling of the bones and irritability.[36] In adults, high vitamin A consumption can result in nausea, drowsiness, hair loss, diarrhea and a loss of calcium from the bones.[36] Fortunately, a reversal of these symptoms occurs once the increased vitamin A usage is stopped[36] With respect to vitamin D, kidney damage and weaker bones has been noted from high intakes of this vitamin.[36] Vitamin K might affect the clotting ability of blood and interact with blood thinner medications. Some research, albeit controversial, has noted higher rates of death associated with vitamin E in excess of 400 IUs a day.[77]

Vitamin A

Vitamin A is called "vitamin A" because it was the very first fat soluble vitamin discovered. While mostly known to help prevent night blindness, vitamin A is also important for maintaining the immune system and proper bone development. As mentioned previously, high levels of vitamin A can become toxic resulting in a number of side effects, the most serious of which is liver damage. Birth defects are also possible if high intakes of vitamin A are used during pregnancy. Multivitamin supplements usually contain beta carotene in place of vitamin A. The body can make vitamin A from beta carotene but do so in a way that avoids its build up to toxic levels. Vitamin A supplements in may increase osteoporosis risk in postmenopausal women.[136] Some research finds high dose vitamin A supplements may increase death rate.[135] Consult physician before using vitamin A supplements.

What is Beta Carotene?

Beta carotene is a member of the carotenoid family of phytonutrients and is found in foods like carrots and sweet potatoes. Many multivitamins contain beta carotene in place of vitamin A because too much vitamin A can damage the liver. The body can convert beta carotene into vitamin A and do so in a way the prevents vitamin A from building up to toxic levels. Some people may also use beta carotene supplements because they think it has anti-cancer or anti-heart disease properties. The rational for this is that beta carotene is found in fruits and vegetables and people who eat these foods tend to get less heart disease, cancer and a host of other illnesses. However, when beta carotene was tested to see if it could protect people from disease, it not only failed but was found to promote lung cancer in smokers and those who worked around asbestos.[80] Several studies have come to the same conclusion and it is generally recommend that smokers and asbestos workers avoid beta carotene supplements. How beta carotene appears to promote lung cancer is not well understood. It is noteworthy to mention that eating foods that contain beta carotene has never been shown to promote lung cancer or any harmful condition. Food contains hundreds of carotenoid and other compounds in addition to beta carotene that probably work together when eaten. The case of beta carotene is something fitness professionals should be wise to remember when discussing high doses of individual nutrients with clients.

Vitamin E

Since its discovery almost one hundred years ago, the fat soluble vitamin, vitamin E (alpha tocopherol), has been not only one of the most popular vitamins but also one of the most controversial. The term vitamin E actually refers to a family of eight related compounds. For example, alpha tocopherol is the type most often found in multivitamins and is the most abundant type in the human body. Other forms of vitamin E include gamma and delta tocopherol. In addition, the vitamin E family also includes compounds called tocotrienols. Most of the interest in vitamin E revolves around its antioxidant capabilities. Antioxidants are molecules that are able to neutralize free radicals, normally produced atoms and molecules which, in excess, are thought to disrupt normal cell operations and contribute to disease. This has lead to the widespread use of vitamin E supplements in an attempt to ward off free radical production and reduce the risk of various conditions like heart disease. Despite its popularity, vitamin E remains controversial with conflicting evidence substantiating its impact on heart disease and other ailments. Some evidence suggests synthetic vitamin E may slow the progression of Alzheimer's disease.[137] Vitamin E does not appear to stop Alzheimer's from occurring.[138] Other, recent data hints that increased rate of death may be associated with high intakes of this vitamin.[80] Because vitamin E has "blood thinning" properties, it could interact with blood thinner medications and as such should be avoided unless prescribed by a physician.

Vitamin D

Vitamin D is a nutrient that is based on cholesterol and is made by the body upon exposure to sunlight. This vitamin is also found in fortified dairy products like milk and yogurt as well. Vitamin D is most often mentioned in conjunction with calcium because it helps the body absorb this mineral. As such, vitamin D can help keep bones strong and offset osteoporosis. Emerging research though suggests that vitamin D may have other uses as well. For example, some research finds that vitamin D may reduce falls in older adults by over 20%.[84] Other studies show similar effects in older adults. Some studies hint that reduced vitamin D may increase the risk of some cancers, multiple sclerosis, and rheumatoid arthritis.[139]

Supplements usually contain vitamin D2 (ergocalciferol) which is plant based or vitamin D3 (cholecalciferol) similar to what we make from sunlight and is thought to be more potent. Our ability to make vitamin D from sunlight tends to decline as we get older. This, and because many seniors may not get outside as much, could accelerate osteoporosis. Likewise, obese individuals may also be deficient.[140] One cup of milk contains about 100 IU of vitamin D. This nutrient is also found in some calcium supplements to enhance calcium absorption. The RDA for vitamin D is 400 IU. When discussing the health benefits of vitamin D, fitness professionals should keep in mind that vitamin D can interact (negatively) with various diseases and medications people may be taking.

Vitamin K

Like vitamin D, the body has a way of obtaining vitamin K internally, thanks to the help of bacteria that live in the human digestive track. Vitamin K is one of the many players in the complex cascade of events that allow our blood to clot when we are cut. Thus, without vitamin K, we might bleed to death if we cut our finger! Aside from this crucial role, other research hints that vitamin K may also be needed to maintain bone strength. Vitamin K supplements are usually not needed by healthy people because of its production by intestinal bacteria. This vitamin is also found in green leafy vegetables. Because of its ability to help blood clot, one side effect often mentioned with respect to vitamin K is its possible interaction with blood thinner medications.

Fat Soluble Vitamins

Vitamin	Selected Function	Sources	Signs of Excess
Vitamin A	Vision	Sweet potatoes, carrots, spinach	Fatigue, irritability, abdominal pain
Vitamin E	Antioxidant	Green leafy vegetables, nuts	Nausea, fatigue
Vitamin D	Calcium absorption	Sunlight, fortified dairy products	Weaker bones, fatigue
Vitamin K	Blood clotting	Intestinal bacteria, soy, green leafy vegetables	Blood clots

The Water-Soluble Vitamins

The water-soluble vitamins include vitamins C and the B complex family of vitamins. The B vitamins can sometimes be difficult to remember because some are referred to by their B vitamin number while others are called by alternate names. For example, vitamin B-12 is often called "vitamin B-12" while vitamin B-9 is usually referred to by its more popular name, *folic acid*. The B complex family of vitamins include vitamin B-1 (also called thiamine), vitamin B-2 (also called riboflavin), vitamin B-3 (also called niacin), vitamin B-5 (also called pantothenic acid), vitamin B-6 (also called pyridoxine), vitamin B-12 (also called cyanocobalamin), vitamin B-9 (also called folate or folacin), and biotin. Inositol (sometimes called "vitamin B-8") is sometimes grouped among the B vitamins however it is made in the body and is not presently thought to be an essential nutrient.

Unlike the fat-soluble vitamins, the water-soluble vitamins are not usually stored in the body for great lengths of time.[36] Unless they are supplied by food or vitamin supplements, deficiencies in many of the water-soluble vitamins become evident after only four weeks.[36]

For the most part, the water-soluble vitamins act as part of enzymes—biological machines which accelerate chemical reactions in the body. Thus, enzymes act as catalysts, by speeding up chemical reactions. For example it might take years for the body to fully digest your last meal if it were not for digestive enzymes.

Energy generating reactions are central to many of the functions of the B vitamins. For example, in the event that insufficient carbohydrates are available, the body can transform protein into glucose to help meet its energy needs. This process is called *gluconeogenesis* and requires vitamin B-6. In addition, B vitamins are needed not only for the storage of fat and glycogen but also for their aerobic and anaerobic breakdown. In spite of their function in energy generating pathways, vitamins do not provide energy directly. The simple reason for this is that vitamins contain no calories (energy).

With respect to exercise, studies generally find that consuming excess water-soluble vitamins (or any vitamins for that matter) does not improve exercise performance, in healthy, well-nourished individuals. This is the reason that most nutrition experts refrain from recommending much more than a multivitamin to athletes and exercisers who eat a healthy diet.

Thiamin

Thiamin is the more recognized name for vitamin B-1. One of the classic thiamin-deficiency syndromes is called *beriberi*—a disease that can lead to paralysis, nerve damage and death. However, thiamin deficiency in the US is rare because flower and grains are usually fortified with this vitamin during processing. Because it is usually consumed by normal, healthy diets, thiamin supplements are usually not needed.

Some people who exercise may supplement with thiamin. The rational for this is that a thiamin deficiency could lead to elevations in lactic acid. Lactic acid is responsible for muscle burning during exercise and also decreases the amount of force that muscles can generate. Thus, lactic acid accumulation can reduce exercise performance. Whether or not supplemental thiamin by those who are not thiamin deficient, can improve exercise performance is not well studied. Good sources of thiamin include lean pork, enriched breads and many fortified breakfast cereals.

Riboflavin

Riboflavin, also called vitamin B-2, was first found in milk in the late 1870s. While required for proper energy production, riboflavin is also needed to help other vitamins like folic acid, niacin and B-6 to work properly. Emerging research also hints that riboflavin may help reduce the incidence of migraine headaches.[85] Riboflavin is a rather delicate vitamin and is easily destroyed by sunlight. This is the reason that many milk containers are not clear plastic. The name riboflavin is a reference to its yellow color. In fact, high intakes of riboflavin are one of the causes for yellow-colored urine that is often observed by people. Riboflavin is usually found in dairy products and green vegetables. Many cereal and grain products are also fortified with this nutrient.

Niacin

Niacin is also called vitamin B-3. Another name that refers to niacin is *nicotinic acid*. The classic deficiency condition associated with niacin is *pellagra*, which results in scaly, dry skin as well as damage to the central nervous system. Pellagra was common in the early 20th century but is relatively uncommon in the US today because many foods are fortified with this vitamin. The body also has the ability to make niacin from the amino acid tryptophan. Alcoholics however, because of their poor dietary habits, are one group where pellagra may still occur.

Niacin normally helps the body carry out many crucial functions required for optimal health such as the making of glycogen and in the breakdown of fat for fuel. High levels of niacin have also been shown to reduce cholesterol and triglycerides as well as boost good cholesterol (HDL) concentrations. Physicians may also prescribe high-dose niacin for this reason. Ongoing research also hints that high doses of niacin may hold promise for staving off cataracts, diabetes and heart disease.[87,88,89]

People with high cholesterol may gravitate to niacin because they want to try a natural treatment before opting to use medications. Keep in mind that high dose niacin is not without risks. For example, some research finds that high intakes of niacin (1-3 g per day) may increase homocysteine by as much as 55%.[86] Homocysteine is thought to also contribute to heart disease risk. Other research finds that niacin can damage the liver and as such is not appropriate for those with liver problems.

Some evidence suggests that vitamin C, vitamin E and beta carotene appear to block niacin's ability to elevate HDL.[90] This may hinder those with cholesterol problems from getting the most out of niacin therapy. High dose niacin may also be inappropriate for those with diabetes because it may elevate blood sugar levels. While definitely needed in small amounts to maintain optimal health, high-dose niacin supplements should only be used by those with medical needs who are under the care of a physician. For healthy persons, there isn't enough evidence to recommend niacin supplements. Good sources of niacin include meats and beans as well as foods fortified with this nutrient.

Pantothenic Acid

Pantothenic acid, also known as vitamin B-5 helps the body burn fats, and carbohydrates as well as extract energy from protein, when it needs to. Pantothenic acid is also needed for the production of acetylcholine, a neurotransmitter (brain chemical) that is needed for all muscle contraction. It is because of its production of acetylcholine that some exercisers may supplement with pantothenic acid. Research to date, while limited, has not observed any significant effect of this vitamin on exercise capacity. Like other B vitamins many foods are fortified with pantothenic acid and deficiency is rare in healthy people eating a well-balanced diet. Foods rich in pantothenic acid include poultry and other meats, legumes and whole grains.

Pantothenic acid is also found in some shampoos. This may be due to the belief by some that the vitamin could prevent hair from turning gray or falling out. This claim appears baseless.

People considering pantothenic acid supplements should take note that only the "right handed" or "d" version can be used by the body. Thus, supplements may list the vitamin as "d-pantothenic acid".

Vitamin B-6

Vitamin B-6, also called, pyridoxine, takes part in over a hundred biochemical reactions that are required for the body to function. For example, the body has the ability to make non-essential amino acids like glutamine and arginine because of vitamin B-6. In fact, Vitamin B-6 is needed to make all of the non-essential amino acids. This vitamin is also required to transform amino acids into glucose, a process called gluconeogenesis. Of all the uses of this vitamin, the one that seems to garner most attention is its ability to lower homocysteine, a chemical linked to the development of heart disease. The vitamins, folic acid and vitamin B-12 also lower homocysteine levels and may appear together in supplements specifically marketed to those interested in heart health. Keep in mind that this is controversial and lowering homocysteine may not necessarily reduce the risk of heart disease.

Another marker of heart disease is an inflammation-related molecule called C reactive protein (CRP). CRP levels tend to rise in response to infections and research is gathering that a chronic elevation in CRP may damage blood vessels in a way that makes them susceptible to the development of artery-clogging plaque. Some research finds that low pyridoxine levels may also contribute to higher CRP concentrations.[91]

Vitamin B-6 is generally considered safe at the RDA. High doses over long periods of time might cause nerve damage and as such should only be used under the supervision of a physician. Good sources of vitamin B-6 include bananas, fish, eggs, poultry and meats.

Folate

Folate, which is derived from a Latin word that means "leaf" (as in leafy vegetables) is also known as folacin as well as vitamin B-9. *Folic acid* is the synthetic form of folate. All terms are usually used interchangeably. Folic acid is needed for the production of DNA, our genetic *blueprint* or *software* program. This fact is related to why folic acid is incorporated to prenatal vitamins—it helps prevent birth defects. Folic acid is also needed to make the hemoglobin portion of oxygen-carrying red blood cells. Thus, deficiencies in folic acid could result in anemia. Folic acid also lowers *homocysteine* which is thought to contribute to heart disease. This vitamin is often added to breakfast cereals and is also found naturally in leafy green vegetables, like broccoli and spinach as well as bananas. One group where folic acid supplements might not be appropriate are those with epilepsy and other seizure disorders. Some research hints that in these individuals, folic acid supplements might enhance seizure rate.[82] The synthetic version of this vitamin (folic acid) is more bioavailable than folate (the natural form). It is for this reason that most multivitamins contain folic acid rather than folate.

Vitamin B-12

Another name for vitamin B-12 is cyanocobalamin. Methylcobalamin is yet another name for this nutrient. Unlike other B vitamins which are found in various amounts in meats and vegetables, vitamin B-12 is only found in meats.

Seniors frequently go to their physician and have injections of vitamin B-12. As we get older we sometimes may have difficulty absorbing this nutrient. Intrinsic factor is a molecule produced by the stomach that helps us absorb vitamin B-12. Conditions such as aging, stomach or intestinal surgery might reduce intrinsic factor production, which in turn limits vitamin B-12 absorption. Reduced stomach acid production as in the case of people who take antacids on a regular basis might also reduce B-12 absorption. Injections of B-12 can bypass this problem. Vitamin B-12 can also be absorbed from the small intestine, although this rout is less efficient.

The liver can actually store vitamin B-12 for great lengths of time, sometimes for many years. In fact, in some cases the body can be so efficient at storing vitamin B-12 that deficiency symptoms may not become evident for 5 years![93] Signs of vitamin B-12 deficiency can include anemia, fatigue, dementia and, if not corrected, irreversible brain damage.[92]

Vitamin B-12 may be used by people who exercise because of thoughts that it enhances energy. Athletes may even get injections of this vitamin in the hopes of supercharging their systems and boosting red blood cell production. Research so far however has not found vitamin B-12 supplements can enhance exercise performance in those who are not deficient in this nutrient.

With respect to health, vitamin B-12 can reduce homocysteine which, as described previously may influence the risk of heart disease. Folic acid and vitamin B-6 also reduce homocysteine levels. Aside from seniors, strict vegetarians (vegans) are also at risk for vitamin B-12 deficiency. While vegetarians can get adequate protein from combining different plant-based foods, they cannot get vitamin B-12 unless they consume meat, dairy or use a vitamin supplement.

Biotin

Biotin is occasionally called *vitamin H* however it is a water soluble vitamin and is generally listed as a member of the B complex family. Biotin helps the body use fats, carbohydrates and proteins and also helps the immune system function. Biotin is stored in the mitochondria, the cellular site of fat burning and when eaten has a very high absorption rate. Thus, deficiency in biotin is unlikely. Biotin is found naturally in cauliflower, peanut butter and soybeans. In addition, bacteria inside the body also make this nutrient. As such deficiency in this vitamin is unlikely.

Biotin is sometimes found in hair products, probably because of a belief by some that it can prevent hair from falling out. This is because hair loss is a symptom of biotin deficiency. Research to date however has not shown that adding extra biotin prevents hair loss in healthy people.

Vitamin C

The other water-soluble vitamin— vitamin C—like many of the B vitamins, is not stored in great amounts in the body. Vitamin C (ascorbic acid) is an *antioxidant* and as such helps protect against cellular damage caused by *free radicals*. It is also indispensable to the proper formation of connective tissue.

Vitamin C may be used by some to prevent colds although research to date has not shown that it can do this. Studies do find, however, that if taken at the first signs of a cold, vitamin C may be able to reduce (by a couple days) the duration of cold symptoms. This is one of the most controversial aspects of vitamin C research and not all research finds that it can reduce cold symptom duration.[94] Regardless of its effects on the common cold, vitamin C does appear to exert influences beyond its curing of scurvy, as mentioned previously. Vitamin C is needed for the production of cartilage and a wearing way of cartilage results in osteoarthritis. Some research finds that vitamin C may help slow the rate of destruction of cartilage.[96] Other research points to vitamin C helping reduce some types of cancer like those of the mouth and stomach.[94] Still other research hints that vitamin C may help keep bones strong.[96] In athletes such as long distance runners and triathletes, a well documented depression of the immune system may occur which can leave the athlete prone to infections in the days following the race. Some research finds vitamin C taken several days prior to a race may be able to bolster the immune system and reduce this risk.[97]

With respect to side effects, vitamin C is known to increase the absorption of iron. Too much absorbed iron may contribute to diseases such as diabetes, heart and liver disease and some types of cancer.[36] In people with a genetic condition called iron overload disease (also called hemochromotosis), too much iron is already absorbed. In these individuals, vitamin C supplements may make their condition worse. It is of the opinion of this author that all people using vitamin C supplements have their iron levels checked. Related to this, some research also suggests that that men with high levels of iron in their blood may be at increased risk of heart disease.[48] This is the reason that some "men's formula" multivitamins do not contain iron.

For those who are going to experiment with vitamin C, keep in mind that we absorb this nutrient better at lower doses. The higher the dose in a supplement, the less of it we absorb.

Antioxidants like vitamin C are very popular among people who are trying to reduce their risk of cancer. While the evidence for this is far from resolved, the use of antioxidant supplements in general by people undergoing cancer treatments like chemotherapy and radiation therapy should be discussed with an oncologist. While more research is needed, some speculate that antioxidants might decrease the effectiveness of chemo and radiation therapies.[98]

What's a Mega-dose?

When discussing vitamins, minerals and other supplements we often hear of the warning not to take high levels of the nutrient in question for fear that doing so might cause unwanted side effects. The often used word to when describing this is "mega-dose". Few people however ever define what a mega-dose is. A mega-dose is an amount that is 10 or more times higher than the recommended dietary allowance.

The Water Soluble Vitamins

Vitamin	Selected Functions	Good Sources	Signs of Excess
Vitamin C	Antioxidant; aids with proper formation of connective tissue	Citrus fruits, broccoli, green peppers, strawberries	Kidney stones, iron overload disease
Vitamin B1/Thiamin	Aids with carbohydrate breakdown	Yeast, pork, beans	Dermatitis
Vitamin B2/Riboflavin	Participates in aerobic metabolism	Beef liver, steak, cheese	Yellow/ orange discoloration of urine
Vitamin B6	Helps with protein synthesis and glycogen metabolism; helps with hemoglobin synthesis	Brewers yeast, lima beans, beef liver	Nausea, vomiting, reversible nerve damage
Vitamin B12	Helps with protein synthesis; helps lower homocysteine; helps with proper red blood cell formation	Meat, fish, milk, poultry	Diarrhea
Niacin	Helps with aerobic and anaerobic metabolism; helps with both fat and glycogen synthesis	Tuna, beef, chicken	Headache, nausea, vomiting, diarrhea, blurred vision, liver toxicity
Pantothenic acid	Helps with aerobic metabolism; helps with synthesis of red blood cells	Egg yoke, yeast, intestinal bacteria	Diarrhea
Folic Acid	Helps with red blood cell formation; lowers homocysteine; lowers neural tube defects	Steak, bananas, salmon	Irritability, excitability, confusion
Biotin	Helps with fat synthesis	Yeast, egg yoke, liver, kidney	None reported

54

Vitamins and Exercise Performance

Multivitamin supplements are the most common form of supplements used by Americans, representing between 70-90% of all products purchased.[36] There is no doubt that the human body requires a wide array of vitamins to function properly. For example, vitamin B_{12} is needed for the proper formation of red blood cells; vitamin C is required for the development of connective tissue (collagen); vitamin D helps calcium absorption. Given their crucial role in health, one might wonder if vitamins enhance exercise performance. Unfortunately this does not seem to be the case. Research since the 1950s has not shown that vitamin supplements improve exercise performance in healthy, well-nourished men or women.[36] In fact, a review of over 90 scientific studies concluded that the vitamin needs of both athletes and non-athletes are rather similar.[17] Some vitamins do take part in chemical reactions involved in energy metabolism. This may have spawned the idea that vitamin supplements provide energy or "pep" during exercise, which is generally untrue. Vitamins do not provide any energy directly because they have no usable calories. Studies of exercising individuals have shown that as physical activity increases, so, too, does the amount of food (and thus, calories and nutrients) that is consumed.[36] Thus, physically active people already tend to be better nourished than non-exercising individuals. For those who wish to have the added "insurance" of a multivitamin, remember that as a general rule, cheaper multivitamins are probably just as effective as more expensive brands.

Natural vs. Synthetic Vitamins

Studies have repeatedly shown that synthetic vitamins, made in the laboratory, are of the same quality as those made in nature. This makes sense, because the molecular structure of both synthetic and natural vitamins are identical and as such the body can't tell the difference.

The case for vitamin E is one classic example often used in an attempt to prove the superiority of natural over synthetic vitamins. It turns out that the body does in fact utilize natural vitamin E better than synthetic vitamin E—and for a very good reason. Some people in the world are left-handed and others are right-handed. The same is actually true for molecules also! Technically, we refer to left-handed molecules as *levorotory* (or L for short). Right-handed molecules are given the name *dextrorotatory* (or d for short). The human body prefers right-handed (d) vitamin E over left-hand (L) vitamin E. Thus, theoretically, natural vitamin E would be composed of all right-handed molecules (i.e. only the d version). Synthetic vitamin E is actually composed of a mixture of both right and left-handed molecules (referred to as "dl alpha tocopherol" on many multivitamin labels) of which we can only use the right handed version. So, in theory, only 50% of synthetic vitamin E can be utilized by the body. It should be noted however, right-handed vitamin E made in the laboratory, is absorbed no differently than right-handed vitamin E made in nature's *laboratory*.

Vitamins as Antioxidants

Many vitamins function in the body as *antioxidants*. Antioxidants are compounds which neutralize highly-reactive, damaging atoms and molecules called *free radicals*. Free radicals combine with other molecules and atoms, and in the process, disrupt normal cellular operation. Free radicals are thought to cause and contribute to a variety of diseases and conditions ranging from heart disease and cancer, to the very aging process itself. The vitamins, A, C and vitamin E are classic examples of vitamins that function as antioxidants. It should be mentioned that the beneficial effects attributed to single antioxidants may be the result of the interaction between several different molecules in food. For example, some studies show an increased risk of lung cancer when smokers take beta carotene supplements.[59] This hints that the beneficial effect attributed to beta carotene may in fact be the result of its interaction with other nutrients in food. This and other facts point to the logic of obtaining antioxidants from food whenever possible. This is sage advice given that we may have not yet discovered all of the nutrients in a given food. If unknown components of food do exist, they may inadvertently be left out of the processing of supplements. Currently, research is undergoing to unravel the effects of various plant chemicals (*phytonutrients*) and the role they play in disease prevention.

The Minerals

The minerals are a group of inorganic compounds, which, like vitamins, are required for the maintenance of health. Minerals are called inorganic because, they do not contain the element carbon. Minerals help with a variety of functions needed for optimal health. For example, iron is needed by every red blood cell in the body and is crucial for the production of hemoglobin, the oxygen carrying component of red blood cells; calcium, while normally only considered when talking about bone strength, is crucial to all muscle contraction as well as blood clotting; the mineral phosphorous is a part of every ATP molecule and magnesium is needed to extract the energy from ATP; no life on earth would be possible if it were not for sodium and potassium which together are fundamental to both the conduction of nerve impulses as well as all muscle contractions.

The minerals can be subdivided into two groups: the *major minerals* – which are required in amounts of more than 100 mg and the *trace* minerals, needed in amounts less than 100 mg.[36]

Boron

The trace mineral boron, used to be utilized as a food preservative. Today boron mostly used as a supplement or is found in supplements alongside other ingredients. Boron is sometimes touted to help a number of conditions but more research is needed to verify most claims. For example, some research suggests that boron may help keep bones strong but the evidence is not as definitive as for that of calcium. Strength trainers used to take boron supplements because of thoughts that it could boost testosterone levels. The research does show that boron may help raise testosterone—if you are an older women who has been put on a boron-deficient diet. Research conducted on healthy men and women who strength train however, has not noted significant elevations in testosterone or strength following boron supplementation. Boron is found naturally in green leafy vegetables, apples, nuts and beans.

Calcium

When most people think of calcium they almost automatically think of bones—and for good reason. Upwards of 99% of the body's calcium is contained in the bones and teeth, where it provides strength, a term technically referred to as *bone mineral density* (BMD). Aside from helping keep bones strong, calcium has other uses as well. For example, calcium is involved in muscle contraction, nerve impulse transmission and blood clotting. There are even calcium-containing adhesive molecules called *cadherins* that act like *glue* and help our cells to stick together!

Another issue where calcium may play a role is weight loss. Some intriguing research has hinted that calcium-rich dairy products, in association with a reduced calorie diet, may help reduce weight.[100] Whether or not calcium supplements produce the same results needs more study.

Because most of the body's calcium resides in the bones and teeth, these places serve as reservoir which the body can draw off of in times when it doesn't get adequate dietary calcium. The problem with this is as the body removes calcium from these areas, they get weaker. Supplemental calcium may be something to consider because research finds that many Americans may not be getting enough of this mineral.

When choosing a calcium supplement, it is important to consider *elemental calcium*. This is the calcium that we use. Different types of calcium have different amounts of elemental calcium. Thus, a 500 mg calcium supplement may not contain 500 mg of elemental calcium. The amount of elemental calcium contained in a supplement may or may not be listed on the product's label. Of all calcium types, *calcium carbonate* has the most elemental calcium (40%). *Calcium citrate* has the next highest (21%). *Calcium lactate* has about 13% elemental calcium and *calcium gluconate* has about 9% elemental calcium. Determining how much elemental calcium contained in a supplement is just a matter of multiplying the milligrams of calcium in the supplement by its corresponding percent of elemental calcium. For example a 500 mg calcium carbonate supplement can be expected to have 500mg X.40 =200 mg of elemental calcium. A 500 mg calcium citrate supplement has 500 x .21 = 105 mg of elemental calcium.

As mentioned previously, long-term lack of dietary calcium can result in *osteoporosis*. Osteoporosis affects more than 25 million Americans with a majority being older women.[38] Osteoporosis results when bone is lost faster than it is made. While traditionally thought of as a condition that only affects older people, osteoporosis is increasingly being viewed as a disease that starts when we are young. This is highlighted by the fact that bone loss begins around the age of 35.[11] The National Institutes of Health (NIH) has recommended that adolescent girls consume 1500 mg of calcium per day.[36] In addition, osteoporosis also affects men, where it contributes to an estimated 10,000 hip fractures each year.[38] Risk factors for osteoporosis include:

1. **Race**. Caucasians and those of Asian decent are at greater risk.
2. **Gender**. Women have a 4 times greater risk of osteoporosis.
3. **Family history**. Risk increases if family members also have osteoporosis.
4. **Age**. Osteoporosis increases as we age.
5. **Early menopause**. Risk increases in those who experience menopause earlier than expected.
6. **Lifestyle behaviors**. Smoking, alcohol abuse, lack of dietary calcium, high intakes of caffeine or salt, lack of exercise and drinking more than 2 cups of coffee per day all appear to increase risk.

Fiber is one of the nutrients known to inhibit calcium absorption. Thus, people on high fiber diets may want to separate fiber-containing meals from calcium supplements by a few hours to enhance absorption. Natural sources of calcium include not only milk and other dairy products but soy, broccoli, boney fish and some mineral waters. Calcium may also added to some commercial orange juices as well.

Chromium

The essential trace mineral chromium is most well known because of its effect on blood sugar. Chromium helps insulin work better and as such may be of help to some type II diabetics by stabilizing blood sugar. Chromium is sometimes called *glucose tolerance factor* (GTF) because of its blood sugar lowering effect although technically this is not true; chromium is part of the GTF molecule but by itself is not GTF. Chromium is often found in weight loss supplements but most research to date does not show it helps.[60] Natural sources of chromium include meats, brewer's yeast, rye bread, fish and tea. For more on chromium see the chapter on dietary supplements.

Copper

The essential trace mineral, copper is needed to make oxygen-carrying red blood cells as well as being required for several enzymes to function properly. For example, copper is needed to make a mitochondrial enzyme (called cytochrome-c oxidase) that is crucial for ATP production. That being said, copper deficiency is rare and supplements are generally not needed. Copper supplements could be dangerous and could damage the liver. The mineral zinc can interfere with copper absorption. This may be something to consider if using zinc to battle colds. Natural sources of copper include meats, nuts, legumes and seafood.

Iodine

The mineral iodine is essential for metabolism. One of the key players in metabolic rate is thyroid hormone, (also called thyroxin). For thyroid hormone to function, it must have iodine. In fact, iodine is so crucial that most of this mineral is stored in the thyroid gland! One classic sign of an iodine deficiency is an enlargement of the thyroid gland, a condition referred to as a *goiter*. Iodine deficiency in the US is unlikely however. Much of the table salt used in US households today is iodized to prevent iodine deficiency. Many processed foods contain salt so adding salt to foods is rarely needed except for personal taste preferences. Besides table salt, good sources of iodine include seafood and to a lesser degree, dairy products.

Magnesium

The mineral, magnesium is involved in hundreds of vital functions including the liberation of energy from ATP, bone formation, muscle function and the making of proteins. Aside from this, some research finds that magnesium may be of help to some diabetics and those with metabolic syndrome by improving insulin sensitivity.[101] Other studies hint that high doses of magnesium may modestly help lower blood pressure in people with hypertension.[102] Lower levels of magnesium appear to elevate C-reactive protein, a marker for heart disease.[103] While obviously crucial for health, magnesium is found naturally in many products like chocolate, green leafy vegetables, whole grains, nuts and legumes. For healthy people, magnesium supplements may not be needed. In high doses, a condition called hypermagnesemia can occur. Symptoms of hypermagnesemia include low blood pressure (hypotension), vomiting and a slowing down of heart rate (bradycardia). These symptoms might start to become evident when magnesium is used above its upper tolerable intake limit of 350 mg a day.

Manganese

Manganese is a trace mineral that's involved in reproduction and proper development of the nervous system. This mineral is also required for the production of superoxide dismutase (SOD) one of the body's natural antioxidants. Manganese synthase, a manganese-based enzyme, is also needed to make the non-essential amino acid, glutamine. Outside of human health, a manganese-containing compound is also sometimes even added to gasoline to boost octane levels. While known to be essential to humans since the 1930s, questions about manganese continue. For example, some research hints that manganese may play a role in offsetting osteoporosis. Deficiencies in this mineral are not likely in the US and supplements are usually not recommended for healthy adults. While unlikely to occur, animal and test tube studies suggest that manganese toxicity might result in the degeneration of the nervous system.[104] Manganese can also hinder the absorption of iron. This could contribute to anemia. Manganese supplements have no known exercise benefit. Foods that naturally contain manganese include shellfish, green leafy vegetables, berries, pineapple, teas, nuts and whole grains.

Molybdenum

The trace mineral molybdenum assists a number of enzymes that help metabolize amino acids. Animal studies suggest that lack of this mineral might impact reproduction, decrease food consumption to unhealthy levels and shorten lifespan. Deficiencies in molybdenum are very unlikely in healthy people and too much molybdenum might interfere with copper absorption. While some research hints that molybdenum-deficient soil might be related to increased esophageal cancer, there is no good proof that molybdenum supplements prevent any form of cancer in humans. Most health experts recommend getting molybdenum from food and not supplements. Foods that naturally contain molybdenum include legumes, peas, milk, nuts and grains.

Phosphorus

Phosphorous is needed by every cell of the body. When delving into phosphorus, one quickly encounters the word phosphate. Phosphate and phosphorus are essentially the same with most of the body's phosphorus occurring in the form of phosphate. For example, readers are probably familiar with the energy molecules, adenosine triphosphate (ATP) and creatine phosphate (CP). In addition to being needed for ATP and CP, both teeth and bones need phosphorus to harden and a lack of this nutrient can weaken bones. While a deficiency in phosphorus is unlikely to occur in those eating a healthy diet, lack of this nutrient can result in muscle weakness, alter the way the heart beats and decrease immunity.

For years, rumors have circulated that soft drinks and other phosphorus-containing beverages might deplete the body of calcium and contribute to osteoporosis. The reason for this speculation is that high phosphorus intake might stimulate parathyroid hormone (PTH) which, in turn, removes calcium from bones. Over time, this could make bones weaker. While in theory, this makes sense, this effect has only been observed under laboratory conditions where people were put on a high phosphorus/low calcium diet.[105] Other research finds that when calcium intake is high (2000 mg/day), high phosphorus intake does not appear to affect bone mineral density.[105] Foods that naturally contain phosphorus include milk, yogurt and other dairy products. Meats are also a good source of this mineral.

Potassium

All life on earth is, in part, made possible because of potassium. Potassium, along with sodium are indispensable for all muscle contraction as well as the transmission of nerve impulses. This transmission of electrical signals is the reason that potassium (and sodium) are also referred to as electrolytes. A lack of potassium (or increase in potassium excretion, as occurs in the case of vomiting or the use of diuretics) can produce a condition called *hypokalemia* and can result in muscle weakness, general fatigue, altered heart function, cramping and abdominal pain.

One of the big areas with regards to potassium is blood pressure. Several investigations have noted lower blood pressures in those with higher potassium intakes. Because fruits and vegetables contain potassium, this is one of the reasons these foods are recommended to people with hypertension. In addition, fruits and vegetables are low in calories which can lead to weight loss. Reductions in weight is also sometimes associated with reduced blood pressure.[106]

Bananas are the classic potassium-containing food with one medium-sized banana providing over 400 mg of this nutrient. However bananas are not the food with the highest potassium content. For example, a medium-sized baked potato supplies over 700 mg of potassium. Other foods that naturally contain potassium include fruits and vegetables, nuts, fish and beans.

Selenium

The trace mineral selenium appears to be essential to human health in a number of ways. For example, selenium is important to the immune system. Related to this, selenium is also required to make an intracellular antioxidant called glutathione peroxidase which helps keep free radicals from getting out of hand. Selenium may show up in supplements alongside vitamin E because of research that finds that these two nutrients work synergistically. Other research suggests that selenium may be of help in reducing the risk of prostate cancer in men. That being said, the usefulness of selenium supplements is controversial and is usually not recommended for healthy people. Like many nutrients, small amounts of selenium appears to be helpful while too much selenium (above the UL for example) might produce symptoms of hair loss, fatigue and a garlic-like odor of the breath.[107] Foods that naturally contain selenium include meats, seafood and poultry.

Sodium

Sodium is one of the body's electrolytes and is partially responsible for the conduction of electrical nerve impulses. Thus, sodium is indispensable not only for nerve signal transmission but all muscle contractions (including the heart!) as well. Too much sodium however is associated with high blood pressure (hypertension). High blood pressure is defined as a consistent resting blood pressure of greater than or equal to 140/90 mm Hg. Increased resting blood pressure over time can damage organs and accelerate heart disease. Besides hypertension, excessive sodium consumption is also one of the lifestyle behaviors associated with osteoporosis.

Sodium is found in many foods and is usually added to processed foods. For example, as a general rule, anything that comes in a box or a can probably has some sodium added to it.

Besides table salt (sodium chloride), which contributes most of our sodium intake, some may be surprised to learn that sodium is also found in soy sauce, monosodium glutamate (MSG), baking powder, sodium saccharin, ketchup, onion salt, garlic salt and some bottled mineral waters.

Some foods are able to list certain health claims on their labels. To be eligible to do this however, they must meet certain standards. For example, foods that are listed as "sodium free" must contain extremely small amounts of sodium (less than 5 mg per serving). Foods that are said to be "reduced sodium" have 25% less sodium than that contained in the original version. Lastly, "low sodium" foods have 140 mg or less sodium per serving. There is no RDA for sodium. People are usually advised to use no more than 2300 mg of salt per day.

Zinc

Zinc is the second most plentiful trace mineral in the body, participating in hundreds of chemical reactions ranging from proper immune function, the sense of smell and taste, wound healing and reproduction to list just a few. Signs of zinc deficiency can include hair loss, dry skin, vision problems, low sperm count, low testosterone levels as well as slowed growth and development.

One of the most popular topics of discussion when it comes to zinc is its impact on immunity. While the studies are controversial in that not all of them show that zinc helps, some research does find that 13.3 mg of zinc gluconate used every few hours beginning at the onset of a cold may help shorten the duration of cold symptoms by a few days.[109] Zinc appears to help the immune system battle colds by interfering with the replication of cold viruses. In other words, by limiting the spread of cold viruses, zinc may help give the immune system more time to mount an effective counter attack. Zinc supplements however do not seem to boost immunity in people who are not sick. In fact, chronic use of zinc supplements might actually weaken the immune system![110]

With respect to exercise, some strength trainers and bodybuilders may supplement with zinc because lack of this mineral has been shown to reduce testosterone levels in men.[108] The effect of zinc supplements on athletic ability, strength and power however has not been adequately studied and a lot of questions remain. Before supplementing with zinc, athletes should determine if they are getting enough of for this mineral to begin with. Zinc is found in many foods and may also be in other supplements athletes may be using. Foods that are good sources of zinc include oysters, fortified breakfast cereals, beef and turkey.

The Major Minerals

Mineral	Dietary Sources	Major Functions	Deficiency	Signs of Excess
Calcium	Milk, cheese, yogurt, dark green vegetables	Blood clotting, nerve transmission, bone strength	Osteoporosis, stunted growth	None reported in humans
Phosphorous	Milk, cheese, meat, fish	Structural component of bone, teeth, cell membranes, ATP	Bone loss. Deficiency is rare	Possible calcium loss from bones
Potassium	Cantaloupe, potatoes, bananas milk, meat	Nerve transmission, muscle contraction	Muscle cramps, irregular heart rhythm	Abnormal heart rhythm
Sulfur	Meats, milk, cheese	Helps with protein synthesis	Deficiency is rare	Very rare. Excess is excreted in urine and feces
Sodium	Table salt	Nerve transmission, muscle contraction	Muscle atrophy, nausea, weight loss	High blood pressure
Chlorine	Fruits, vegetables, salt-containing food	Helps maintain pH of body	Unlikely to occur if chloride containing foods are consumed	High blood pressure
Magnesium	Green leafy vegetables, coffee and tea	Muscle contraction, extraction of energy from ATP	Growth problems	Depression, nausea, diarrhea

The Trace Minerals

Mineral	Dietary Sources	Major Functions	Deficiency	Signs of Excess
Iron	Lean meats, green leafy vegetables	Oxygen transport	Weakness, fatigue, infections	Iron overload disease
Fluorine	Drinking water, seafood	Helps with bone formation	Increased cavities	Nausea, vomiting, abnormal heart rhythm, death
Zinc	Meats, wheat germ	Protein synthesis	Growth problems	Fever, vomiting, diarrhea
Copper	Meats, drinking water	Needed for iron use	Anemia	Nausea, vomiting and diarrhea
Selenium	Seafood, meats, grains	DNA repair, immune functioning	Anemia	Hair and nail loss, nausea, vomiting
Iodine	Vegetables, iodized salt	Component of thyroid hormone	None reported in humans	Very high intakes inhibit thyroid activity
Chromium	Meats, nuts, cheese, whole-grain bread	Involved in glucose and energy metabolism	Decreased ability to use glucose effectively	Some evidence that chromium (chromium picolinate) may cause DNA damage

Recommended Vitamin and Mineral Intakes

Vitamin	Adult RDA	Adult AI	Adult UL
Vitamin A	Men:600 µ Women: 700 µ		10,000 IU (3,000 µ)
Vitamin D	Up to age 50: 200 IU Age 51-70: 400 IU Over 70: 600 IU		2000 IU
Vitamin E	22 IU natural vitamin E or 33 IU synthetic vitamin E		100 IU synthetic / 1500 IU natural
Vitamin K		Men: 120 µ Women: 90 µ	Not established
Vitamin C	Men: 90 mg Women: 75 mg		2000 mg
Thiamin (B-1)	Men: 1.2 mg Women:1.1 mg		Not established
Riboflavin (B-2)	Men: 1.3 mg Women: 1.1 mg		Not established
Niacin (B-3)	Men 16 mg Women 14 mg		35 mg
Pantothenic Acid (B-5)		5 mg	Not established
Pyridoxine (B-6)	Men: up to age 50: 1.3 mg Men over age 50: 1.7 mg Women: to age 50: 1.3 mg Women over 50: 1.5 mg		100 mg
Folate (vitamin B9)	400 µ		1000 µ
Cyanocobalamin (B-12)	2.4 µ		Not established
Biotin	30 µ		Not established

Minerals	Adult RDA	Adult AI	Adult UL
Boron	Not established		20 mg
Calcium	To age 50: 1000 mg Over age 50: 1200 mg		2500 mg
Chromium	Men to age 50: 35 µ Men over 50: 30 µ Women to age 50: 25 µ Women over 50: 20 µ		Not established
Copper	900 µ		10 mg
Iodine	150 µ		1.1 mg
Iron	Men: 8 mg Women up to age 50: 18 mg Women over age 50: 8 mg		45 mg
Magnesium	Men to age 30: 400 mg Men over 30: 420 mg Women to age 30: 310 mg Women over 30: 320 mg		350 mg
Manganese		Men:2.3 mg Women: 1.8 mg	11 mg
Molybdenum	45 µ		2 mg
Phosphorus	700 mg		Up to age 70: 4,000 mg Over age 70: 3,000 mg
Potassium	Not established	4.7 g	
Selenium	55 µ		400 µ
Sodium	Not established		2300 mg
Zinc	Men: 11 mg Women: 8 mg		40 mg

As can be seen from the table, for some nutrients there is no RDA. For example, an RDA has not been established for potassium. Nutrition experts generally however usually recommend 3000-3500 mg a day of this mineral be consumed in food.[93] Boron, once popular among some fitness enthusiasts because of a mistaken belief it could raise testosterone levels, also has no RDA.

What are Phytonutrients?

The prefix *phyto* means *plant*. *Phytonutrients* are not vitamins or minerals but rather components of fruits, vegetables, grains and teas which are thought to play a role in health. Currently there is no RDA for phytonutrients and no deficiency-syndromes associated with a lack of these compounds are known to exist. Emerging evidence however is finding that phytonutrients (phytochemicals) may play a role in health and the prevention of various diseases. For example, some evidence suggests that various phytonutrients may act as antioxidants, and as such, may protect the body from syndromes such as cancer and heart disease. Examples of phytonutrients include the *carotenoids, anthocyanins* and *isoflavonoids* to name a few. Hundreds of phytonutrients are currently known to exist. Studies show that people who consume a diet rich in fruits and vegetables tend to be healthier overall than those who do not. These observations have prompted research to uncover which nutrients might be responsible for food's protective effects. Unfortunately the research on phytonutrients is still in its infancy. For example, as mentioned previously, studies have found that smokers who use beta carotene supplements have a *higher* rate of lung cancer compared to non-smokers.[80] This is just the opposite as is observed when people eat foods containing beta carotene. Lycopene a phytonutrient found in tomatoes is sometimes used by men because of research hinting that it might help reduce prostate cancer. However most of the research on this nutrient involves eating tomatoes. It is possible that fruits, vegetables, grains and teas protect against disease because of the interaction of several thousands of phytonutrients all working in concert with each other. If this is true, then consuming large amounts of single phytonutrients, like lycopene or beta carotene, might not work the same as consuming fruits and vegetables—and may result in outcomes quite opposite from what was expected.

Nutrition Terminology

When discussing vitamins, minerals and nutrition in general, readers soon encounter several terms and acronyms which bear discussing here:

International Units (IU). Some drugs and vitamins are measured not in milligrams or grams but rather in international units. For example, the potency of vitamin E is often listed in international units (for example 400 IU). Confusion often arises when people try to covert between IUs and a more common unit of measure like milligrams. International

Units are a measure of the potency of a vitamin or drug while milligrams, grams etc. are a measure of a compounds weight. Conversion factors do exist to help nutritionists translate IUs to milligrams, which may be needed in certain clinical situations. For example, to convert from IUs to mg of dl alpha tocopherol (synthetic vitamin E), multiply the IUs by 0.45.

GRAS. The letters GRAS stand for *generally recognized as safe* and is a term used by the FDA and other nutrition agencies to denote compounds that have been in the food supply before 1958. Thus substances listed as GRAS either have a long track record of safety or have scientific evidence that finds they are safe for human consumption. Nutrition research is always continuing. Under law, compounds that are currently listed as GRAS may in fact be de-listed as evidence contrary to their safety comes to light.

Bioavailability. This term refers to how much of a nutrient is available to be absorbed by the body. Some nutrients like protein are highly absorbable while others like the mineral chromium are less well absorbed.

Daily Value (DV). Daily values are listed on food labels and are based on the RDA. They represent suggested nutrient intake levels that all persons can use, regardless of age or gender. The Daily Values however are based on a 2000 calorie a day diet. As a rule, a healthy 2000 calories a day diet should provide daily values of 1200 calories of carbohydrate, 600 calories from fat and 25 grams of fiber.

RDA. Recommend Dietary Allowance. The RDA is the average daily intake of a nutrient that is sufficient to meet the needs of most healthy persons of a particular age and gender. There are many RDAs. For example, there is an RDA for children, adults and pregnant women. In an attempt to make the RDA more applicable to all people, a new set of terms was created which all come under the heading of the dietary reference intakes (DRI), which are defined below.

Dietary Reference Intake (DRI). This is a term that many people may not be aware of and is used mostly in academic settings. The dietary reference intake is a term designed to be more encompassing than the RDA. In fact, the DRIs actually contain the recommended dietary allowance. There are four DRI values:

1. **RDA:** the recommended dietary allowance mentioned above

2. **Estimated average requirement (EAR).** This value is the amount used to meet the nutrient needs of half of healthy persons of a particular age group and gender. The EAR is one of the numbers that helps with the establishment of an RDA

3. **Adequate Intake (AI).** For some nutrients an RDA has not yet been determined. When no RDA is available, a nutrient is assigned an Average Intake (AI) number. These values are approximations of how much of a nutrient is thought to be adequate for healthy individuals.

4. **Upper Tolerable Limit (UL)**. Too much of any nutrient might produce undesirable side effects. The Upper Tolerable Limit (UL) is the uppermost amount of a nutrient that can usually be tolerated by people without side effects. Intake that exceeds a nutrients UL, enhances the chances that side effects might occur. This is not to say that side effects will definitely occur but rather that the *potential* for side effects is increased at levels above the UL.

Chapter 7

Dietary Supplements

Those in the fitness and nutrition field will undoubtedly be asked about dietary supplements at some point in their career. Currently tens of thousands of dietary supplements are on the US market. While it is beyond the scope of this book to review all supplements, this chapter provides a basic review of some of those which the fitness professional may be asked about. For expanded, reviews of these topics and over 100 other popular supplements, read the book *Nutritional supplements: What Works and Why,* available at www.Joe-Cannon.com.

What are Dietary Supplements?

Dietary supplements refer to a wide range of substances that are meant to *supplement* a healthy diet. The official definition of dietary supplements stems from the Dietary Supplement Health and Education Act of 1994 (called, *DSHEA* for short). According to this act, a dietary supplement is defined as:

> "a product (other than tobacco) intended to supplement the diet that bears or contains one or more of the following dietary ingredients: a vitamin, mineral, amino acid, herb or other botanical OR a dietary substance used to supplement the diet by increasing the total dietary intake OR a concentrate, metabolite, constituent, extract, or combination of any ingredient described above AND intended for ingestion in the form of a capsule, powder, softgel, or gelcap, and not represented as a conventional food or as a sole item of a meal or the diet AND is labeled a dietary supplement".

This definition is the basis for all of the tens of thousands of supplements on the US market today. All dietary supplements sold must adhere to these guidelines. Products that fail to meet the criteria of this definition cannot be legally called a "dietary supplement".

Occasionally the Food and Drug Administration (FDA) takes action against companies that market products that either do not adhere to DSHEAs supplement definition or those which make specific claims that the product may act in a manner similar to a drug, which is illegal, under current US law. Sometimes this action is in the form of a warning letter cautioning a company to curtail what the FDA deems as inappropriate marketing practices (like making drug claims). In other instances, the FDA may actually seize a product and ban its sale because of evidence that the product is inappropriately packaged, is adulterated with other substances or is dangerous.

Sometimes these actions scare people into thinking that the government is trying to restrict the sale of supplements. Indeed, occasionally, editorials even appear in some newspapers and magazines alleging that this is so. The odds of this happening however are quite remote. DSHEA has been the law of the land since 1994. In addition, evidence continues to accumulate that some supplements, when used properly, have beneficial effects on health.

What is Peer-Reviewed Research?

Peer-reviewed research is the best type of research. To have a study that is peer-reviewed means that before the study was published in a scientific journal, it was first reviewed by other competent scientists (the "peers") whose job is to look for mistakes or flaws in the experiment. Any errors in research that are discovered during the peer-review process must be fixed before the study is accepted for publication. Essentially, having a study published that is peer-reviewed means that you did your homework and dotted all of your I's and crossed all of your T's. The scientific journals in which peer-reviewed research is published are generally not found in the magazine section of your local supermarket. You must subscribe to them and subscriptions may cost hundreds of dollars a year! Articles appearing in popular magazines are generally not peer-reviewed, but they sometimes are based on peer-reviewed research studies.

Examples of peer-reviewed scientific journals:

• Journal of the American Dietetic Association
• Journal of Nutrition
• Pharmacotherapy
• Journal of the American Nutraceutical Association
• International Journal of Sports Nutrition and Exercise Metabolism
• Medicine and Science in Sports and Exercise
• Journal of Strength and Conditioning Research

Amino Acid Supplements

Amino acids are often called the building blocks of proteins because many amino acids linked together form proteins. Some people take amino acids supplements in order to enhance muscular strength and development. While consumption of amino acids may indeed contribute to muscle growth, supplements that contain amino acids however may not be the best course of action. When ingested, there is no guarantee that amino acids in the supplement will be used to help build muscle. The body may incorporate the amino acids from the supplement into growing muscles or it may use them to make enzymes that help keep wax out of your ears! Another problem with taking just one or a few amino acids is that it does not provide as broad of a spectrum of amino acids as eating food does. Amino acid supplements also tend to be more expensive than food.

Amino acids do have different properties and research hints that some of them may have usefulness that goes beyond their incorporation into muscle proteins. For example, marathon runners may use supplements that only contain branch chain amino acids (BCAA). These amino acids—specifically leucine, isoleucine and valine—are thought to compete with and maybe impede the entry of tryptophan (another amino acid) in to the brain. The body needs tryptophan to make serotonin, a brain chemical that is involved in fatigue. Thus, by reducing tryptophan via BCAA supplements, runners might, in theory, stave off fatigue during exercise. BCAAs may also reduce the body's reliance on glycogen during exercise and thus extend the time before glycogen exhaustion sets in. Currently though the effectiveness of this strategy is mixed with research finding that it either may help or not help. Some evidence hints that BCAAs may stimulate the release of insulin from the beta cells of the pancreas.[111] As such BCAA supplements might interact with medications used by diabetics. For athletes who are considering BCAA supplements but who are on a budget, 3 ounces of tuna fish supplies the body with ample supply of these amino acids.

Androstenedione

Androstenedione ("andro") is not really a dietary supplement but rather a hormone made within the adrenal glands.[20] Andro is sometimes popular among strength trainers because it is one chemical step from the anabolic hormone testosterone. Thus, the rationale behind using androstenedione is that it will lead to greater testosterone levels, which in turn might promote enhanced muscular development. However, clinical studies to date have failed to show that androstenedione enhances muscular growth, strength or athletic performance.[8,43] In fact, some research finds that it may raise estrogen levels in men! Because it is a hormone, androstenedione is not without risks. Emerging evidence suggests that androstenedione may lower HDL ("good" cholesterol) levels. This might in turn raise the risk for heart disease. Pro-hormones like androstenedione should be used with caution because of a lack of proof of their long-term safety.

Black Cohosh

Black cohosh is an herb which grows in North America and was first introduced to early European settlers by the American Indians. These days the main reason people use black cohosh is to relieve menopause symptoms. The scientific names for black cohosh are *Actaea racemosa* and *Cimicifuga racemosa*.

Some studies have found that black cohosh may be of modest help at reducing hot flashes and other symptoms associated with menopause and premenstrual syndrome (PMS). However, not all research finds that it works. In addition, most studies finding positive results with black cohosh agree that at least a few weeks of continued use is needed before any reduction in menopausal symptoms is noticed. Because of its apparent ability to reduce some symptoms of menopause, it has been generally believed that black cohosh has estrogen-like activity. However this is still being investigated and debate continues as to how black cohosh works.

Osteoporosis is a disease where bones become brittle and break easily. Estrogen is needed to help keep bones strong. Because black cohosh is thought to possess estrogen-like qualities, some feel this herb may help osteoporosis. Currently, this is speculation and black cohosh should not be used as a substitute in place of osteoporosis medications prescribed by a physician.

Carnitine

Carnitine is sometimes popular among those trying to lose weight. Carnitine is one of the molecules that is involved in moving fat to the mitochondria where it can be broken down ("burned") for energy. Because of this, some speculate that additional dietary carnitine may help the fat-burning process by bringing even more fat than normally possible to the mitochondria to be utilized. While in theory this might sound plausible, most of the research on carnitine supplements to date finds this is not so.[13,57] Carnitine is generally considered safe in healthy people.

Chromium Picolinate

Chromium is a trace mineral. *Picolinate acid* (which is part of chromium picolinate) is a natural metabolite of the amino acid, tryptophan. One of the roles of chromium is to help regulate blood sugar.[26] Studies of young, growing animals have hinted that chromium picolinate may be effective at reducing body fat as well as improving muscle mass. However, several human studies have failed to show this effect.[60] At least one study has shown that chromium picolinate may promote weight *gain* in young overweight females.[25] Other investigations of chromium ranging from college football players to overweight military personal have found neither reductions in body fat or enhancements in muscle mass following chromium supplementation.[36] Based upon the preponderance current evidence, chromium picolinate does not appear to contribute significantly to muscular development or fat loss in healthy humans.

Since the 1990s there has been some concern that high levels of chromium picolinate might cause mutations in the genetic material (DNA) of humans which, in theory, might lead to diseases like cancer.[112] Conclusive human research on this topic is lacking. In fact, most of the evidence on this issue stems from test tube studies and animal research. This is very different than research on humans. Thus, this area is very controversial. Adding to the controversy is that not all research finds chromium picolinate is harmful. It is important to make the distinction between chromium itself and picolinate acid. The research to date generally points to picolinate acid as a possible culprit behind DNA mutations. The mineral chromium is safe.

Creatine

Creatine is a natural product made in the body and is also found in meats and fish. Studies dating back to the 1960s have found that the use of creatine supplements may improve strength and power. As such, creatine is sold as a dietary supplement touted to improve strength and power in those participating in very high intensity activities like powerlifting, bodybuilding and sprinting.[60] When ingested, creatine, becomes *phosphocreatine*, a molecule which is able to regenerate ATP during times when ATP must be made extremely fast. As such, creatine acts like a *supercharger* for ATP production. Faster energy production rates translate into a longer ability to sustain a high intensity activity and an enhanced capacity to recuperate between bouts of exercise. These characteristics allow an athlete to sustain a high intensity stimulus for a longer period of time—which stimulates the body to make more muscle proteins (myosin, actin etc.) that help muscles grow stronger. Putting this another way, the longer the muscles are under stress, the stronger they become.

Creatine is of little benefit to those participating in long-duration or low intensity activities like jogging, triathlons, hiking or yoga. Likewise, creatine supplements are probably of little help to those engaged in moderate-intensity resistance training programs. In other words, creatine would be of more help to those lifting a weight for between 1 repetitions to 10 repetitions as opposed to somebody who lifts for 15 to 20 reps.

Creatine and Sports

Creatine Might Help	
• Powerlifting	• Bodybuilding
• Football	• Shot putting
• Sprinting	• Javelin throwing
• Boxing	• Martial arts

Creatine Might Not Help	
• Triathlons	• Marathons
• Group aerobics classes	• Circuit strength training
• Horse racing	• Bicycling
• Jogging	• Hiking

Loading creatine—a practice whereby people take a lot of creatine for the first week (20-25 grams a day usually)—does not seem to be needed. Research shows that a month of using only 3 g of creatine a day puts as much creatine in the muscles as does 20 grams for a week.[129]

With respect to side effects, no serious negative side effects have been observed with creatine to date. Rumors of abdominal cramping and muscle/tendon tears resulting from creatine supplementation are possible but have generally not been observed in research. The most consistent side effect from creatine supplementation is an increase in body weight, due most likely to increased water retention.[60] People with kidney problems are usually cautioned against using creatine for fear that it might overtax already wakened kidneys. Creatine might also be detrimental to those with liver problems. Many different creatine products are on the market. The type that has been used most in research is *creatine monohydrate.*

Echinacea

Echinacea is generally regarded the world over as an herb that can help the body combat colds and other infections. Specifically, some research finds that echinacea may be able to reduce the duration and severity of colds by roughly 10% and 30% when taken at the very start of cold symptoms.

Three different species of echinacea are known to exist: *Echinacea angustifolia*, *Echinacea pallida* and *Echinacea purpurea*. Of these, the last species (echinacea purpurea) has most of the evidence. How echinacea stimulates the immune system is still a mystery and the active ingredients in the plant are still under investigation. Also unknown is how much is needed? With respect to infections, one thing does seem clear; echinacea does not prevent colds when taken every day. In fact, regular use of this herb may actually depress the immune system![29]

With respect to side effects, because of its possible stimulation of immune system cells, echinacea is not recommended for those with autoimmune diseases such as rheumatoid arthritis, lupus or type I diabetes. Likewise the use of echinacea is controversial in those with HIV infection because it might worsen symptoms.[29] It is also noteworthy to mention that not all research shows echinacea is effective at helping battle colds.

Ephedra

Ephedrine is a drug derived from the plant *ephedra* which mimics the action of adrenalin (epinephrine) in the body. Another popular name for ephedra is *Ma Huang*. Some studies have concluded that ephedrine use can promote small amounts of weight loss, probably an average of about two pounds more per week than when not using ephedrine.[49] Because the weight that is lost is small, ephedra is often combined with other agents such as caffeine and aspirin, which are said to boost its effects.[18]

Side effects from ephedrine use can include elevated blood pressure and heart rate, as well as strokes and seizures.[18] Psychosis has also been reported following the use of ephedrine.[18] Ephedra can raise blood sugar levels and as such may be inappropriate for diabetics. Because ephedrine can elevate heart rate and blood pressure, it is not appropriate for those with heart or blood pressure disorders or those with a family history of these diseases. At least 100 deaths have been reported to the FDA that have been associated with the use of ephedrine-containing products.

Individuals who wish to use ephedrine containing supplements should be strongly urged to consult their physician prior to using such products. Those who experience an adverse reaction after taking a dietary supplement can report their reaction to the Food and Drug Administration by calling 1-800-FDA-4010. Ephedra is controversial in that studies show it appears to work; however it carries some significant health issues when used inappropriately.

Possible Ephedra Side Effects			
• Dizziness	• Restless	• Nausea	• Vomiting
• Headache	• Anorexia	• Difficulty urinating	• Rapid HR
• Flushing of skin	• Hyperthermia	• Insomnia	• Psychosis
• Elevated BP	• Irritability	• Heart failure	• Death

Glucosamine Sulfate

Glucosamine sulfate is a compound made naturally in body and plays a role in the proper formation of cartilage.[19] Specifically the sugar glucose and the amino acid glutamine unite to form glucosamine sulfate. Studies dating back to the 1970s have noted that glucosamine sulfate, might help reduce the pain associated with osteoarthritis, the most common type of arthritis that results when the cartilage cushioning between bones wears away.[19] Because of this, glucosamine sulfate is a popular remedy among those seeking a natural alternative to arthritis drugs. Most glucosamine research generally finds that it helps about as much as aspirin and that it takes about two months before a reduction in pain is noticed. How glucosamine seems to work is not well understood and some studies show it might not work. While glucosamine does not seem to re-grow joint cartilage, some evidence does hint that this supplement may help by slowing the progression of osteoarthritis.[116]

Glucosamine supplements are often combined with another compound called chondroitin sulfate. Whether or not glucosamine plus chondroitin work better than glucosamine alone is controversial. It should be stressed the glucosamine only appears to work for osteoarthritis. Glucosamine does not help rheumatoid arthritis or other forms of this disorder.

With respect to side effects, glucosamine sulfate appears to be generally safe. Occasionally questions as to whether glucosamine raises blood sugar levels surface but this effect has not been well documented in humans. People using blood thinner medications should be cautious however. Both glucosamine and chondroitin may interact with blood thinner medications. For more information, read my book *Nutritional Supplements: What Works and Why*, available at my website, www.Joe-Cannon.com.

Whole-Food-Based Supplements

Whole-food-based dietary supplements are essentially fruits and vegetables in capsule form. These dietary supplements are based on the premise that individual nutrients (like vitamin C, for example) are *fragmented*—that is, they only provide one component of what is required for health. Advocates of this philosophy content that since nutrients to work in conjunction with other nutrients, taking individual vitamins and minerals may be an inefficient road to optimal health. Thus, according to some proponents, dietary supplements based upon entire foods may be superior because food has not only vitamins and minerals but in addition phytonutrients, which are also thought to promote health. Currently, most of the published clinical research on these products is on a whole-food supplement called Juice Plus +®. Whole-food-based dietary supplements are not a substitute for food but, given that many Americans do not consume a "wide variety" of fruits and vegetables everyday, this may be a option for those who wish to add more fruit and vegetable extracts to their diets.

Supplements and the Fitness Professional

Despite advertisements to the contrary, the words *natural* and *safe* do not mean the same thing. Fitness professionals should investigate supplements for side effects, drug interactions, quality and any proof that substantiates a product's advertised claims before discussing them with clients. While there is little doubt that some dietary supplements may hold promise for improving health and wellbeing as well as some aspects of exercise performance, they should never been seen as a shortcut. All dietary supplements are designed to *supplement* a healthy diet—not replace it. As always, good nutrition is the foundation of all exercise and wellness programs.

Fitness professionals should also check with their place of employment and determine what supplement policies are in place before discussing any product with clients or members. Because of the past controversy surrounding some supplements (i.e. ephedra), some fitness facilities may strictly prohibit staff members from discussing supplements with clients or club members. It is also noteworthy to mention that some personal trainer liability insurance carriers will not protect fitness professionals from lawsuits brought about as a result of dietary supplements.

There is little doubt that personal trainers, group aerobics instructors and other members of the fitness industry have been seen by the vitamin and supplement community as avenues to further market their products to the public at large. This is capitalism and networking and there is nothing wrong with this. Good nutrition and exercise go hand-in-hand. Fitness professionals should remember however that their first duty is always to their clients and what they advocate is a reflection on them and the quality of their services. Before using or discussing any dietary supplement, questions should always be asked. The questions listed below can be used as a guide to help when researching dietary supplements.

Dietary Supplements: Questions to Ask Yourself

---

1. Is there any *published* peer-reviewed research showing that the product works?
2. If yes, is the research on the *product* or the *ingredients* of the product?
3. Are the levels of ingredients in the product the same as that used in research?
4. Who was the research conducted on (men, women, bacteria, animals)?
5. If the product is promoted for weight loss, how was weight loss determined in research? Underwater weighing is the most accurate method available.
6. Is the research published as a full fledged scientific paper (i.e. not an abstract)?
7. How many peer-reviewed studies on the product have been published that find that it does what its reported to do?
8. Have any side effects or drug interactions been observed in research?
9. If the answer to question #8 is yes, what are the side effects and drug interactions?

Supplement Buzz Words

Advertisements for supplements tend to use a host of words to convey to the public that a product is quality. Popular buzz words used in advertisements include the following:

- Clinically proven
- Patented
- Amazing
- Technology
- Breakthrough
- All natural
- Modulate
- Bioactive
- Innovative
- Anti-aging
- Quick
- Easy
- Miracle
- Toxin
- Effortlessly

Words and phrases like these show up frequently in health, fitness and nutrition advertisements. In reality, all of these terms are vaguely-defined and to the trained professional mean very little. Remember words like these should never take the place of quality, peer-reviewed research that's published in clinical journals.

Chapter 8

Metabolism

Everybody it seems likes to talk about metabolism. Some people have "slow" metabolisms while others have "fast" metabolisms. The problem is that few people understand what metabolism is. That is what this chapter is all about.

Right now as you read these words, millions of chemical reactions are occurring. Some of these chemical reactions are resulting in something being created while others are undoubtedly breaking things down. Thus, one way to define metabolism is to think of it as the sum total of all the building up and tearing down processes in the body. The building up metabolic processes are called *anabolism*. It is from the word anabolism that we get the term *anabolic*. The classic example of an anabolic reaction is the building of new muscle tissue although even the forming of new cells that line your digestive track is anabolic. At the other end of the spectrum are the tearing down metabolic processes which are referred to as *catabolism*. It is from the word catabolism that the term *catabolic* is derived. In some circles catabolism is a *bad* word. This is understandable considering that the breakdown of muscle that occurs from disuse or disease is a catabolic reaction. It's important for the fitness professional to recognize that all catabolic reactions are not bad. For example, the digestion of food is a catabolic reaction. The breakdown of ATP, our ultimate energy molecule and the breakdown of glycogen, our stored carbohydrate reserve, are also a catabolic reactions.

Another way in which to understand metabolism is to define it as the number of calories that are consumed ("burned") at rest. This definition gives rise to the terms *resting metabolic rate* and *basal metabolic rate*. Resting metabolic rate (or RMR) is is the speed at which we burn calories in a resting state and accounts for approximately 70% of our daily caloric expenditure.[5] Basal metabolic rate (or BMR) is the minimum number of calories needed to keep us alive. You are at your basal metabolic rate when you are sleeping. While often used interchangeably, technically RMR and BMR are not the same thing; basal metabolic rate is lower than resting metabolic rate.

Factors that Impact Metabolism

It turns out that the rate at which we burn calories can be affected by several factors. For example, as a rule, men tend to have slightly higher metabolisms than women. Thus, *gender* is a factor which impacts metabolism. Other factors that influence metabolism are as follows:

- **Age.** Metabolism tends to decrease as we grow older. As a rule resting metabolic rate drops by about 2% to 5% per decade after age 25.[27] This is one of the reasons why people gain weight as they get older.

- **Climate:** Metabolism tends to increase in colder environments. This makes sense given that our body wants to maintain an internal temperature of about 98.6 degrees F. Lowering the outside temperature essentially makes us fire up the furnace!

- **Thermic effect of food:** The thermic effect of food (TEF) refers to the fact that it takes calories (energy) to digest and metabolize food. Thus, eating will raise metabolism however, not very much. One of the reasons protein is sometimes used by those trying to lose weight is that it raises metabolism more than carbohydrate or fat does. This is because protein has a slightly higher thermic effect than the other two macronutrients.

- **Activity level:** Exercise can raise metabolism.

- **Hormones:** Hormones are chemical messengers. While thyroid hormone (thyroxin) plays a role in metabolism, so, too, do other hormones like testosterone, growth hormone, and insulin. Some hard-core bodybuilders may even inject insulin! This is because besides helping put sugar in cells, insulin also helps us utilize amino acids. The problem however with non-diabetics injecting insulin is that, when injected, the body stops making its own insulin. Upon stopping insulin injections, the body may even go into a rebound diabetic state! Another problem is that no evidence shows that injecting insulin by non-diabetics improves muscle mass, strength or athletic performance.

- **Body composition:** Muscle is a metabolically active tissue and consumes more calories at rest than fat. Muscle mass alone contributes to approximately 22% of RMR.[5] Thus, the more muscle a person has on his or her body, the greater the resting metabolic rate (RMR) tends to be. While controversial, some have estimated that every pound of muscle burns somewhere between 20 and 80 extra calories a day.

Exercise and Metabolism

One of the main reasons people exercise when trying to lose weight is to boost metabolism. Exercise can be subdivided into aerobic and anaerobic activity. Both types are important to do but impact metabolic rate differently. For example, minute by minute, we tend to expend (burn) more calories with aerobic exercise than during resistance training. Stated another way, a 150-pound man burns approximately 648 calories per hour during aerobic exercise but only 432 calories per hour during strength training.[5]

Another way to differentiate between aerobic and anaerobic activity is the length of time that each elevates metabolism. Aerobic exercise, has its biggest impact on metabolic rate during the activity. This can easily be seen from the example in the last paragraph. However, metabolism tends to return to normal resting levels one or two hours after cessation of the activity.[133] Resistance training, on the other hand, may lead to elevations of metabolic rate that can last 16 or more hours after exercise.[5] That being said not all research shows that resistance training significantly raises RMR.[133] Other factors that might also contribute to this after-strength training elevation in metabolic rate include the amount of muscle used during exercise, the weight lifted (the volume of weight also), the rest periods between sets and the fitness level of the individual. Alterations in these factors may contribute to the conflicting results of exercise on RMR.

Dieting and Metabolism

Studies have shown that dieting can result in a lowering of both resting and basal metabolism.[36] In fact, severe calorie restriction may lower RMR by as much as 45%.[36] This reduction in metabolic rate actually makes sense when one considers that the body doesn't *understand* why less food is being eaten. For all the body knows, a global catastrophe might be responsible for eating less. It doesn't know it may live just down the street from a convenience store! The body only knows that less calories are being consumed and it does the only thing it can to stay alive—slow the rate of fuel (calorie) consumption. In the event of a global catastrophe, a slower metabolic rate means a person might live long enough find more food. While staying alive is obviously a good thing, the slowing of metabolism that accompanies dieting can sabotage ones weight loss goals by making it harder to lose weight. This is one of the reasons that most diets don't work in the long run.

Another problem with diet-induced reductions in metabolic rate is that the body may start to *circle the wagons*, so to speak. In other words, the body may actually begin to digest its own muscle tissue to stay alive. This can lead to an atrophy of muscle size and strength. As many fitness professionals are aware, when a muscle cell is lost, it never returns. Humans unfortunately do not seem to be able to make new muscle cells. All that can be done is to build up what is left.

Related to the more familiar type of atrophy described above is a process that some fitness professionals may not be aware of—*sarcopenia*. Sarcopenia refers to an age-related loss of muscle tissue. In other words, sarcopenia tends to occur as we grow older. More specifically, *sarcopenia*, is an age-related loss of type II muscle cells. The body has essentially two types of muscle cells – *type I* and *type II*. Type I fibers are slow twitch fibers and are used during endurance activities. Type II are designed for strength and power and there are two subtypes: *Type IIa* fibers are fast twitch muscle cells and are able to produce muscle endurance as well as generate a good amount of strength. *Type IIb* muscle fibers, are also fast twitch fibers but are completely anaerobic muscle cells that produce the most strength and power. While sarcopenia normally occurs as one ages, long-term, low calorie dieting, coupled with inadequate protein and nutrient intake might accelerate this process. The reason for this is that the body, in an attempt to keep itself alive, performs a sort of *triage*, assessing what can stay and what can be broken down to maintain life processes. Unfortunately, as we age, we exercise less.

Also, in the case of dieting, energy levels might fall to a level preventing one from maintaining their fitness level. The body, in these instances, may not *think* it needs its type IIb fibers any longer and begins breaking them down. If left, unchecked, this scenario would eventually have a detrimental impact on one's quality of life, years later.

Obviously, for many people, the process of sarcopenia described above is a worst case scenario and a few weeks of doing most diets is unlikely to have a significant effect on the process. For fitness professionals working with older adults, however sarcopenia is a real possibility. Older adults tend to eat less food—and less protein. They also tend to not exercise. Of those who do exercise, very few strength train. While the process that leads to sarcopenia is still a mystery, it does appear that two of the best ways we have to reduce its impact it to eat well and exercise regularly.

Estimating Metabolic Rate

There are several ways to estimate metabolic rate. For example, one popular method calls for multiplying the body weight of males by 11 and that of women by 10.[27]

Males	RMR = Body weight X 11 cal/lb
Females	RMR = Body weight X 10 cal/lb

The numbers 10 and 11 are used because it is estimated that a man's body needs about 11 calories per pound to maintain its basic operational needs. A woman's body needs about 10 calories per pound. For example, a 200 pound man needs about 200 X 11 = 2200 calories a day to maintain current metabolic rate. A 200 pound woman needs about 2000 calories a day (200 X 10). This method however is not highly accurate. Usually people ask about metabolism because they want to lose weight. Another equation that can be used is to multiply ones desired body weight by 13. For example, if one were 160 lbs and wanted to be 140 lbs, 140 X 13 = 1820 calories. In theory, eating 1820 calories in this example should help one eventually reach their 140 lb goal. Another, even easier, way is it to simply reduce the number of calories one eats. Generally, eating 250-300 less calories per day should promote weight loss in most people. Fitness professionals should be conscious not to decrease calorie intake too much, lest they significantly decrease metabolic rate which in turn might negatively impact weight loss. According to some, consistently losing more than ½ lb per week might lower metabolic rate.

As for exercise, *at least* 60 minutes of moderate intensity exercise 3-5 days that burns about 2000 calories per week is usually recommended for weight loss.[133]

Chapter 9

Eating Disorders

Fitness professionals will undoubtedly come across people who have issues with eating. This is especially true for those counseling clients about nutrition. While this chapter is not all-encompassing, the main goals are to review some of the more common conditions and provide insights as to how to best assist individuals in coping with this problem. Eating disorders are serious conditions and taken to extremes can be fatal. The fitness professional should never view him or herself as a client's only resource but rather seek out other competent professionals within the healthcare continuum, like registered dietitian, psychologists and physicians when faced with issues that he or she feels may be beyond their capabilities.

Female Athletic Triad

Female athletic triad is a phrase first coined by the American College of Sports Medicine (ACSM) to describe a syndrome of three distinct but often related medical disorders that are observed in adolescent and young adult female athletes. The syndromes comprising female athletic triad are:[3]

1. *Disordered* eating patterns
2. *Amenorrhea*
3. *Osteoporosis*

These three issues are of growing concern, especially due to the pressure on adolescent girls to maintain what they think is an "ideal" body weight. In women who develop female athletic triad, excessive exercise or inadequate nutrition affect the ovaries, which respond by reducing estrogen output. Reduced estrogen levels, in turn, cause bone loss and accelerate the rate of osteoporosis. This can have a profoundly detrimental impact on quality (and quantity) of life years later.

Estrogen also plays a role in protecting women from heart disease. Thus, an issue not often mentioned is that a lack of estrogen as a result of amenorrhea might also increase the risk of a heart attack in younger women. Amenorrhea may also affect cardiovascular health years later after their sports careers are over. The consequences of amenorrhea may not be taken seriously by young athletes who think of themselves as invincible and do not comprehend its possible far reaching consequences. In fact, fitness professionals should not be surprised by competitive athletic women who are not overly concerned with their lack of menstruation. Amenorrhea however is a serious concern and women should be referred to their physician/gynecologist who can best monitor them over time.

Who's at Risk of Female Athletic Triad?

Women who participate in sports, strive for thinness in hopes of performing better or look better while performing their sport are at risk for female athletic triad. These women are overly concerned with weight, food, and body shape. Athletic activities where female athletic triad may be observed include but are not limited to, gymnasts, jockeys, swimmers, race car drivers, female professional wrestlers and bodybuilders, fashion models, marathon runners and triathletes. Female athletic triad may also be common in college female athletes whose education is partially or fully funded because of athletic scholarships. It is important to note that it is not only elite athletic females at risk for this condition. Any physically active female may be at risk of developing female athletic triad.[3]

Dealing with Female Athletic Triad

While there are no easy answers, fitness professionals working with young athletic females should strive to instill in their clients a healthy body image. Negative comments about body weight should be avoided. Coaches who instill a negative body image in a female athlete as a way coax her to lose weight are wrong.

Currently, the incidence of female athletic triad is not fully known; however, studies suggest that anywhere from 15-62% of female athletes have some form of disordered eating.[21] Given these statistics, young girls should be encouraged not to be affected by what the media depicts as the "perfect body". Women should be made aware of the fact that what the media often depicts as *healthy* is often unrealistic and is helped by airbrushing and other camera tricks. The young female should also feel comfortable enough to communicate her feelings to both her parents and physician. While often a touchy issue, inquiring about menstrual cycles may also help identify those with this condition. The intervention of a registered dietician or sports nutritionist who has experience with female athletic triad may also be required to help the athlete get back on track.

Anorexia Nervosa

Anorexia nervosa is the refusal to maintain an appropriate body weight for one's age, height and gender. Individuals with anorexia nervosa have an intense fear of gaining weight and a preoccupation with dieting and being thin. [36] Basically, people with this condition don't eat very much. In spite of being thin, people with anorexia nervosa view themselves as being overweight. To combat the perceived fatness, individuals will often subject themselves to large volumes of exercise to reduce their perceived fatness. With weight loss comes the eventual stopping of menstruation (amenorrhea) described previously. While anorexia nervosa is present in between 1 to 2% of the general population of America, between 6 and 20% of those afflicted with the syndrome die as a result of various factors including suicide, heart disease and infections. [36]

An aspect of this condition not often talked about is oral health. While on the surface, the health of the gums, teeth and oral cavity may seem trivial when compared to other outcomes described above, the preservation of a healthy oral cavity is nonetheless an aspect of long-term health maintenance. Here's why: Research has linked gym disease and tooth decay to the development of heart disease. Some evidence suggests that people with gum disease have higher levels of C reactive protein (CRP) a compound that appears to impact the risk of heart disease. Thus, a lack of proper nutrition coupled with an intake of nutrient deficient foods might not only lead to bone loss and gum disease but increase heart disease risk as well.

Signs and Symptoms of Anorexia Nervosa

- Refusal to maintain appropriate body weight for one's gender, age and size
- Extreme fear of gaining weight in spite of being very underweight
- Altered body image, i.e. the perception of being fat even though they are underweight for their age, gender and height
- The absence of at least three consecutive menstrual cycles

Bulimia Nervosa

The name bulimia nervosa makes reference to the almost insatiable appetite observed in those afflicted with the syndrome.[36] Bulimia is characterized by frequent occurrences of binge eating (usually at night) which is almost always followed by vomiting.[36] Bulimia is a somewhat more frequent manifestation than anorexia nervosa in that bulimia is seen in 2 to 4% of adolescents and adults. The majority of individuals afflicted with this syndrome are female.[36] Following binge eating, individuals with bulimia tend to starve themselves by fasting and may also use laxatives or water pills to aid in the expulsion of ingested food.[36] Individuals with bulimia may also exercise excessively as a way to rid themselves of calories. Bulimia may occur in those who are overweight or normal weight.

Signs and Symptoms of Bulimia Nervosa

- Excessive concern with body weight and body composition
- Frequent gains and losses in weight
- Visits to bathroom following meals
- Recurrent instances of binge eating, usually in secret
- Binge eating followed by periods of not eating and/or vomiting
- The use of laxatives or water pills to expel food or the use of excessive exercise to expend calories
- Irregular menstrual cycles

Muscle Dysmorphia

Women usually figure prominently in most discussions on eating disorders and body image problems with men often being neglected. This is unfortunate because men can suffer from these concerns as well. Although not technically classified as an eating disorder, one example of a not often mentioned male-issue is muscle dysmorphia. Sometimes, muscle dysmorphia is used interchangeably with a more popular term, called the Adonis Syndrome however technically, they are not the same. The Adonis Syndrome can refer to a number of body image or physical conditions that men may want to change or take steps to avoid. This can range from hair loss, plastic surgery, sexual potency issues and body fat reduction to name a few. Muscle dysmorphia however is specific in its reference to the intense desire to have bigger muscles. Symptoms of muscle dysmorphia may include excessive exercise (sometimes exceeding 2 hrs a day) that takes priority over other activities like job, family and hobbies, avoidance of social situations and a preoccupation with how attractive their body looks. They may also experiment with steroids or dietary supplements reputed to increase muscle size and strength. In a nutshell, men with muscle dysmorphia see themselves as small and weak even though they appear big and strong to everyone else. Some individuals with muscle dysmorphia may have eating disorders (about 30%), experience anxiety and depression over their body image and may take part in radical types of diets. In this respect, muscle dysmorphia shares some similarities to anorexia described previously. In fact, muscle dysmorphia used to be called "reverse anorexia" in some medical circles.[122] Men experiencing muscle dysmorphia may also wear layers of clothing to look bigger or clover up their perceived smallness. Injuries, resulting from overtraining syndrome may also be common in these individuals. While this condition may occur in any sport, it appears most common in sports like bodybuilding where muscle symmetry is an issue.

Symptoms like those described above are general and could probably describe a number of people, including even some fitness professionals. By themselves some of these signs may be perfectly normal although when they are combined with depression, steroid abuse, low self esteem, anxiety and/or suicidal thoughts, or when their preoccupation with exercise as a way to improve appearance is at the expense of family, friends and occupation, then counseling with a qualified professional may be in order.

Signs and Symptoms of Muscle Dysmorphia

- Preoccupation with how their body looks
- Excessive time spent working out
- Exercising at the expense of family, friends and hobbies
- Perception of being small or weak even though they are not
- Continuation of exercise even when injured
- Layering of clothing to appear bigger
- Steroid abuse
- Eating disorders

Chapter 10

Client Assessment

For many fitness professionals, especially those who are new to the field, the idea of what needs to be done when first meeting with a new client can be a scary thing. Most fitness professionals have a working understanding of weight lifting technique, target heart rate, calories, protein, fat, carbohydrate and related issues, but deciding what needs to be completed before an effective exercise and nutrition program is designed can be a mystery. This chapter will deal with issues surrounding how to assess the current fitness and nutrition status of clients. The goals for this chapter are to better prepare the fitness professional to deal one-on-one with new clients and help them make their first sessions with new clients run as smoothly as possible.

The Initial Interview

The initial interview is the first meeting a fitness professional will have with a new client. This time can be used to gather valuable information as well as to demonstrate to the new client your proficiency and professionalism. The initial interview should be conducted in a private area, such as an office or cubical if possible. This is not only because the client may be divulging sensitive information such as personal contact information but also because it may help assuage uneasiness that the client may feel during any testing that may occur. Taking circumference or body fat measurements in a public area is one of the fastest ways to make a new client feel not only uneasy but also demonstrate to him or her the unprofessional setup of your operation. While this may not be an issue for fitness trainers who travel to people's homes, for health clubs that are space-limited, this can be a difficult obstacle to overcome. Health clubs however that wish to improve profit margins by incorporating premium services such as nutrition counseling or personal training should take steps to dedicate a private area devoted specifically to this purpose.

The initial interview also gives the fitness professional and new client an area to get to know each other and engage in conversation. While on the surface, this may seem secondary to the main goals of the initial interview, this time together can aid in the gathering of valuable information. Take body language for example. It is sometimes stated that only 20% of a spoken sentence is verbal with the other 80% non verbal. Body language like posture, making eye contact, firmness of handshake, folding of arms and other non-verbal cues can help the fitness professional get an idea of where their clients are in terms of their motivational level and other aspects of their personality. Sitting timidly in a chair, not making eye contact or removing coats when indoors may be signs that the person is depressed or feel that they cannot do anything to improve their circumstances. Maybe they have tried every diet on the market and have worked in the past with a fitness professional without any progress? Maybe you are their last hope! Recognizing a persons subconscious non-verbal signals can be a remarkable asset because it will help you to better put their fears and anxieties to rest and form a bond between you both.

Fitness professionals should also provide their personal contact information such as cell phone number and/or email address. This is also a good idea for trainers working in a health club setting. Business cards made on any home computer can make this easy to do. Providing this information will help the client schedule sessions as well as facilitate easy cancellation of training sessions if an emergency arises. Phone numbers should have voice mail so clients can leave a message. If communicating via email, it is in the fitness professionals' best interest to provide their clients with a *professional*, easy to spell email address. This can be something as simple as "yourname@yahoo.com". Pornographic or otherwise suggestive email addresses are inappropriate and is one of the fastest ways to make a bad impression on a new client.

The initial interview is also a good starting place to begin collecting general and medical history information. Much of this information is easily obtained by having the new client complete a medical or health history questionnaire, one of which is provided for your convenience in the Appendix section at the end of this book. Basically, all health history forms contain into the following sections:

Personal Contact Information

Information such as name, address, phone number, email address, emergency contact name and phone number and the client's primary care physician is listed here. All personal and medical history data that is collected should be kept private. Fitness professionals should refrain from specifically discussing a client's personal or private information with other colleagues in a way that would allow for the client to be identified. In addition, the client's specific conditions etc. should not be discussed in public settings like restaurants. Personal trainers should keep all of their client's information in an organized filing system such as in a filing cabinet that has the ability to be locked. This is especially important if the records are being maintained in a hospital setting such as a hospital-based fitness center that may be subject to specific privacy regulations.

Personal Medical History

This section provides information regarding the clients' personal medical status. Questions to ask in this section can and should include those regarding diseases and syndromes experienced by the client as well as questions about surgeries and injuries. Other questions can include those pertaining to cholesterol levels, blood pressure and cigarette smoking habits. Whether or not they are currently exercising should also be inquired about.

Fitness professionals, who encounter clients with serious medical issues like heart disease, diabetes, cancer, etc., should refer them to their primary care physician and obtain a written approval note from that physician prior to working with the individual. This serves not only as an extra measure of safety for the individual but also may help the fitness professional down the road in the event of litigation. Obtaining a note from a qualified medical professional can also been seen as a marketing opportunity. Physicians can be difficult to schedule a meeting with during the day because they are busy with patients, paperwork, and other tasks that make demands on their time. By referring high risk clients back to their physician prior to training, opens up an opportunity for physician to get to know you and your services better. More importantly, doing so also speaks volumes to medical professionals about the level of competency and care you provided to their patients.

Conditions that Warrant a Physician's Permission Prior to Exercise

• Heart disease	• Chest pain at rest	• Emphysema
• High blood pressure	• Chest pain during exercise	• Pregnancy
• Kidney disorders	• Diabetes	• Cancer
• Prior heart attack	• HIV/AIDS	• Asthma
• Pacemaker	• Morbid Obesity	• Sedentary lifestyle
• Heart surgery	• Early death of parents	• Stroke

Family Medical History

Most medical history forms will have a section that inquires about the health of immediate family members. This information may in turn shed light on issues which the client may encounter in the future. For example, information that a client's parents suffered from osteoporosis may help the fitness professional better counsel the client on strategies to minimize the risk of osteoporosis in his or her own life. It can also be seen as another opportunity to identify high risk individuals as well. Research finds that those whose mother, sister or daughter died suddenly before the age of 65 or father, brother or son who suddenly passed away before the age of 55 may be at an increased risk of early death from heart disease.[2]

Medications

Personal trainers are generally not physicians or pharmacists. While some very good books and websites do exist which can educate personal trainers on medications, diseases and other conditions, asking about medication usage is not to prompt the fitness professional to attempt to analyze the effects of medications. Rather, the goal should be seen as another opportunity to identify high-risk individuals. Clients using medications for serious medical conditions like high blood pressure (hypertension), diabetes, heart disease, kidney disorders, cancer, etc., should be referred back to their physician prior to working with the individual. A release note from their physician should also be obtained for your records as well.

Dietary Supplement Use

Dietary supplements are very popular among people, so it is likely that clients will be using them or have used them in the past. While some supplements may in theory help reduce disease risk factors, many supplements lack peer-reviewed clinical evidence. Knowledge of a clients' dietary supplement usage may allow the fitness professional to better educate their clients on well balanced nutrition habits. An excellent resource on this topic is *Nutritional Supplements: What Works and Why,* available at www.Joe-Cannon.com.

Fitness History

Given the relationship between exercise participation and reduction of various disease states, as well as weight loss, the fitness professional may want to inquire about this aspect of health as well. Knowledge of someone's exercise likes and dislikes can also can help the personal trainer design an effective exercise program for their clients that is not only enjoyable but also addresses any specific needs they may have. For example, clients indicating that they play a particular sport or activity give the personal trainer the opportunity to incorporate movements that may strengthen muscles that can help them play their sport better as well as strengthen muscles that may be prone to injury.

PAR-Q

PAR-Q stands for Physical Activity Readiness Questionnaire and is a one-page form that can help the personal trainer identify people (ages 15-69) who may not be ready to begin an exercise program. Essentially, the PAR-Q asks a series of simple questions. Answering yes to any question on the PAR-Q means that the person may have a significant medical issue and should be referred to their physician before exercise training begins. Questions usually asked on the PAR-Q include:[2]

1. Has your doctor ever said that you have a heart condition and that you should only do physical activity recommended by a doctor?
2. Do you feel pain in your chest when you do physical activity?
3. In the past month, have you had chest pain when you were not doing physical activity?
4. Do you lose your balance because of dizziness or do you ever lose consciousness?
5. Do you have a bone or joint problem that could be made worse by a change in your physical activity?
6. Is your doctor currently prescribing drugs (for example, water pills) for your blood pressure or heart condition?
7. Do you know of any other reason why you should not do physical activity?

The questions of the PAR-Q can be incorporated into a section of a standard health history questionnaire or be a separate form altogether. The actual PAR-Q form can be viewed online by connecting to an Internet search engine like Google™ and typing in the phrase "PAR-Q and You". Some people reading these words may be the owners of health clubs. By having all new members complete the PAR-Q before joining can effectively screen for many high-risk individuals and provide an added layer of protection for those who wish to start an exercise program.

The Liability Waiver

Fitness professionals, whether working at a health club or self employed, should have all new clients sign a standard liability waiver. The liability waiver can offer some legal protection in the event that litigation occurs. Fitness professionals should have am attorney create the waiver. Clients should not only sign the waiver but understand it as well. Liability insurance should also be a must for all fitness trainers as well.

The Client/ Trainer Agreement

The client/trainer agreement is a form that essentially outlines the responsibilities of the fitness professional as well as those of the client. It is here that the fitness professional will list information that he/she feels is necessary and important. Items that could be listed here include, dressing appropriately, when fitness testing will occur as well as what will be tested, cancellation policy and training package duration. Some trainers may use the form as a motivational tool. In other words, some people may be more likely to continue with personal training and make progress toward their goals if they sign their name to a form. This form is not legally binding and as such is used at the trainers discretion.

Setting and Achieving Goals

Before walking in the door for their first meeting, new clients will undoubtedly have many goals that he or she will like to accomplish. The fitness professional should make certain that these goals are realistic and attainable. For example, the goal of losing 30 pounds in one month is not realistic or healthy and is probably not attainable for most people. Large goals should be broken up into smaller, more manageable and realistic goals. Thus, the fitness professional and the client should work together to modify goals which may by unrealistic in the short term. Breaking large, lofty goals, into smaller, more manageable chunks will help prevent the client from getting discouraged over time.

Fitness professionals are also fitness educators. One way in which personal trainers can educate their clients that goes beyond proper exercise and nutrition habits is by teaching people the power of writing down their goals. Studies show that when people write their goals down on paper that they are more likely to achieve those goals in the long run. Some health clubs actually have *goal sheets* which new clients complete to help the trainer get an idea of what the person wants to accomplish. The problem with this however is that everybody will probably have very similar goals (e.g.

lose weight, tone up, etc.) and the more the trainer sees the same thing over and over, the less likely he or she may pay attention to it. Having said that, lets now discuss a better way to list goals.

When setting goals, clients should be encouraged to write their goals out and to be as specific as possible and give the reasons why they want to achieve those goals. Simply writing "I want to lose weight" is vague and probably isn't going to be adhered to. A better written goal is "I want to decrease my weight by 20 pounds because it will help reduce the pain I feel in my knees and help lower my blood pressure" Obviously, goals written like this may require some thought on the part of the client, so assigning this task as *homework* may be needed. This idea of homework can actually be a good thing because when clients sit down in private they may really start to think about the real reasons why they want to achieve their goals. When doing this exercise, encourage the client to be as honest and frank as possible and to hold nothing back. Reassure them that nobody will ever view what they have written. This is crucial because what they will probably write will be their private, innermost thoughts and feelings. By having people commit to writing their goals in this way helps them take ownership of those goals. In essence, they have taken a small step. By committing to a small step like this, studies show that they are more likely to take the bigger step of achieving their goals!

Once you have their goals and have broken them down, where needed, into attainable short and long term attainable objectives, fitness professionals should review the goals on a regular basis with their clients. This also should occur in private. Fitness professionals should sit down with the client and with clipboard in hand ask questions such as "what have you done over the past week to achieve your goals?" and "what have been your set backs, if any?". All answers should be written down and techniques to address overcoming any obstacles to progress should be addressed. Progress should also be reinforced to help spur the client toward the continuation of goal achievement.

Nutrition Assessment

Prior to giving specific nutrition advice, the fitness professional should have clients complete a personal nutrition assessment. A nutrition assessment is simply a written record of what foods a person consumed over a specified time period. One of the most common methods is to have clients write down what they consumed over a 3 day period of time. This is sometimes called a *three-day food diary*. Information to report in the food diary can include:

- What food was consumed?
- Amount of food that was consumed?
- What time was the food was consumed?
- Was the person hungry when food was consumed?
- How were they feeling (e.g. happy, sad etc.)?

This information will give valuable insights into not only the eating habits of clients but may also provide information into what provokes them to eat. For example, it may be noticed that when a client is sad or depressed he or she eats large amounts of high calorie foods. This information may allow the client to take steps to avoid high calorie foods during times of stress or depression. It's important that the client eat normally and not substitute foods which he or she feels the fitness professional would want them to eat. It's also important that the days listed on the three-day food record represent *typical* days. Days that are not typical, include special events like weddings, etc., and should not be included in the three-day food log.

Clients should strive to be as specific as possible as to the types of foods they are eating. For example, listing "soda" is not as specific as listing "12 ounces of diet orange soda". "One slice of bread" is better reported as "one slice of whole wheat bread". Being specific can be a double-edged sword, however, because people who become overly precise may begin actually measuring their food. This could lead to an underreporting of what is actually consumed. Related to this, people should not weigh the food they eat because this also may lead to underreporting. An abbreviated sample of a food journal created with Microsoft Excel is as follows:

Sample Three-Day Food Diary

Time of Day	Place Food was Consumed	What was Consumed	Amount Eaten or Calories	Feelings
Day 1				
Day 2				
Day 3				

Obviously, the journal depicted above is a very simple example of what can be made on anyone's home computer. Other more sophisticated templates may be found on various websites. Yet another alternative to making a food journal yourself is to reach out to pharmaceutical representatives for assistance. Many drug companies have weight loss medications and pharmaceutical representative have a wide assortment of items that they routinely give to doctors and other health care professionals to help advertise these products. Pocket-sized food journals are most likely among those items that fitness professionals may obtain for free. Keep in mind that these pocket journals will likely bear advertisements for a weight loss medication. Some fitness professionals may not advocate such medications however these food journals will be professionally made and can be an asset for those looking for something portable. Another alternative, especially for those who want to continually track food consumption over longer periods of time are software programs that can be purchased and downloaded onto PDAs or home computers. These programs can be quite sophisticated and have areas for imputing exercise and foods eaten.

It is important to make clear to clients that the purpose behind the three-day food journal is not to make them feel guilty about what they are eating but rather, to help give themselves insights into what they are eating. While writing down what was eaten is probably not something that a person should do forever, occasionally completing a three-day food journal may provide the individual with feedback on their eating choices and help keep them on track for the long haul.

Obstacles to Progress

Many clients will undoubtedly encounter areas which prevent their goal attainments. For example, some clients may find it difficult to abstain from purchasing high calorie, high fat foods when shopping at the supermarket. Clients may not be aware of the fact that supermarkets are designed in a way that keeps consumers in the stores for as long as possible. The longer they are in the store looking for something, the more items they come in contact with and more they are tempted to buy (see the chapter on *supermarket self defense)*. To help combat this, the fitness professional may suggest that the client eat prior to shopping to nullify urges to purchase what is not needed. Going to the supermarket with a shopping list can also help keep people on track. By having a shopping list, people know exactly what they need and spend less time roaming around aimlessly. Personal trainers may also want to accompany clients to the supermarket or hold seminars for clients on how to read food labels.

Record Keeping

The nutrition professional should maintain up-to-date records on all clients. This begins with the very first meeting and continues throughout the association with the client. Each meeting with the client should be documented and placed in the client's folder so as to facilitate easy retrieval if needed at a future date. Information which should be recorded at each meeting should include:

- The date of the meeting
- Issues which were discussed during the meeting
- Areas where the client is having difficulty as well as areas in which he or she is excelling
- Areas for future follow-up—e.g. asking the client to present the 3 day food journal at your next meeting

In addition, the nutrition professional should record other valuable information at regular intervals such as the client's weight, percent body of fat, body circumferences and BMI. These measurements do not have to be taken at every meeting but rather at intervals spaced far enough apart so that a picture of the client's progress can be tracked over time.

The client should not be made to feel uncomfortable during these measurements. Rather, personal trainers should reinforce the fact that these calculations are part of the *big picture*, which is the ultimate improvement of the health of the individual. Along with these measurements, the nutrition professional should also record other improvements/obstacles to progress which the client may volunteer during routine conversations. Examples may include reductions in clothes size, reductions in cholesterol levels or improvements in performing activities of daily living such as walking up stairs, etc.

While some may choose to keep track of clients on their computers, it is highly recommended that hard copies of client meetings be kept on paper as well to minimize the loss of data which may occur during a computer mishap. Client data on the computer should also be backed at regular intervals to minimize the loss of information.

Body Composition Analysis

Fat can be divided into two different reserves: *essential fat* and *storage fat*. Essential fat represents the fat that is needed for the body to continue to carry out normal life processes. Essential fat consists of that in the liver, spleen, bone marrow, muscles, intestines and the central nervous system [36]. Essential fat represents only about three percent of the total body fat in men and about 12% of the fat in women.[36] Storage fat is all fat reserves above and beyond essential fat. Average percentages of body fat for college-age men is 12% to 18% and 16%-25% for college-age women.[27] Obesity is defined as body fat in excess of 25% for men and 30% for women.[27] Many studies find that disease risk increases as body fat increases. Research also notes that the location where fat is stored also plays a role on disease development. For example men tend to store much of their fat around their abdomen. This fat distribution pattern is linked to greater rates of heart disease than that seen in females, who tend to store much fat around the hips and thighs.

Body Fat Percentages		
	Men	**Women**
Average	12% - 18%	16% - 25%
Obese	> 25%	> 30%

Body composition refers to the relative amounts of fat and muscle on the body. While many individuals may use a household scale to estimate their weight, a scale usually only provides one raw number (total body weight) that does not distinguish between muscle and fat. While the scale can help keep people on track, other tools are also available that can provide deeper insights into a persons body composition. Some methods are, of course, better than others and all have their drawbacks. The fitness professional should have an understanding of the different methods available to assess body composition in order to help his/her clients reach their maximum potential while reducing the incidence of a variety of diseases. Because of this, the following overview of various popular body composition analysis techniques is offered.

Body Typing

This is an older method that attempts to classify people into one of three types: *ectomorph*, *mesomorph* and *endomorph*. The ectomorph is said to be thin and have a hard time gaining weight. Endomorphs are said to be at the other end of the spectrum, being round, and having a hard time losing weight. Mesomorphs are said to have a muscular build and narrow waist. Problems with this type of analysis include the fact that it doesn't consider percent body fat and not everybody fits into these classifications; some may be composites of each. Also, classifying people as specific body types may provide people with a *crutch* that prevents attainment of goals.

Height–Weight Tables

Height-weight tables assess body composition based on gender and the size of one's frame. Like scales, height-weight tables do not assess the amount of body fat a person has. Rather they compare people to an "average" person. Problems abound when using these tables for body composition analysis. For example, many professional athletes are considered overweight when assessed with height-weight tables.[36] Because of error and because other, better methods exist, the fitness professional should not rely solely on height-weight tables to determine body composition.

Body Mass Index

The body mass index (BMI) is calculated from the equation:

$$\text{Weight (in kilograms)} \div \text{height (in meters}^2)$$

That is, one calculates BMI as the weight of a person (in kilograms) divided by the person's height (in meters squared). This is written in the form "kg/m^2". For example, if a person weighed 200 lbs. and was six feet tall, his BMI would be calculated the following way:

1. Convert pounds to kilograms. Since there are 2.2 lbs in a kilogram, 200 lb. ÷ 2.2 = 90 kilograms.

2. Convert the person's height to meters squared (m^2). Since the person is six feet tall and since there are three feet in a meter, the person is two meters tall. Now square this amount (that is, 2 meters X 2 meters) to get $4m^2$

3. The persons BMI is 90 kg / $4m^2$ = 22.5 kg/m^2

BMI is sometimes useful as a quick assessment of a person's risk of disease because obesity-related health problems increase as BMI increases over 25 kg/m^2 for most people.[2] According to current guidelines, a BMI of 25-29 kg/m^2 is classified as "overweight" and a BMI of over 30 kg/m^2 is considered "obese". A BMI of 40 or more is classified as "extremely high" or being at extremely high risk of obesity-related diseases.[2] While BMI offers a quick and relatively easy way to assess a persons' body composition, it does have its limitations. For example, like the height-weight tables described previously, many professional athletes would be classified as "obese" via BMI determination. Looking at this from another point of view, BMI does not differentiate between muscle and fat. Two people can be the same height and weight and thus have the same BMI yet one person may have a body fat percentage of 10 percent while another may be 35%. In addition, there is a ± 5% error when determining body fatness from BMI.[2] Thus, caution should be used when labeling a person overweight or obese from the calculation of BMI alone.

Body Mass Index Values	
BMI (kg/m2)	Meaning
Less than 18.5	Underweight
18.5 - 24.9	Normal weight
25.0 -29.9	Overweight
Greater than 30	Obese

Circumference Measurements

The advantage of circumference measurements is that it is quick and easy and only requires a tape measure that the fitness professional uses to measure the circumferences of various body areas. This information can be plugged into equations to estimate body composition or can be used to track changes over time. Alternatively, the measurements themselves can be used by themselves as a check of progress. The major disadvantage of this type of body composition analysis is that it gives little information about the amounts of fat and muscle a person has. Nevertheless, for the fitness professional working with morbidly obese individuals, this method offers a way to track changes while at the same time not making the client feel overly self-conscious. The following table lists areas that are commonly measured for girth.

Circumference Measurements

Area	Where Measurement is Taken
Neck	Distance around the neck
Waist	Most narrow part of the torso
Abdomen	At the umbilicus (belly button)
Hips	Maximal circumference of the buttocks
Thighs	Largest circumference of the thigh
Calf	Maximal circumference of calf
Chest	Around the mid-sternum, just above the nipple line
Upper arm	Around the midpoint of the upper arm
Forearm	Maximum girth of the forearm

When measuring limb circumferences, do so in the straightened, un-flexed position. This will provide information on the limb's resting circumference. While some may choose to measure only the right limbs, both sides can be measured if desired. Fitness professionals working with very obese people should keep in mind that they may be unable to measure abdominal circumference because of excess abnormal fat. Those wanting to avoid possible embarrassing situations may wish to not measure this area in morbidly obese individuals.

From information of circumference measurements, it is possible to calculate the *waist to hip ratio* (sometimes abbreviated as *WHR*). The waist to hip ratio is often used to estimate the degree of abdominal obesity, which is seen as a greater risk for heart disease than fat relegated to the hip and thigh areas. In other words, as WHR increases, the risk of obesity-related diseases also is increased.[2] A waist to hip ratio of greater than 0.95 for adult men or 0.86 for adult women indicates that individuals are at greater risk of developing diseases associated with being overweight.[28]

It is important to remember that professional athletes may have a very high WHR when they are in fact at low risk for obesity-related diseases. Thus, the use of WHR should be used as a general guideline and not as the definitive measure of obesity. In other words, it is possible to have a high WHR and not be obese at all.

Alternately, waist circumference alone can be used to estimate disease risk. Men with a circumference greater than 40 and women greater than 35 are said to be at increased risk of obesity-related diseases. In fact, research suggests that waist circumference alone is a better predictor than BMI.[131]

Skin Fold Analysis

Another way to estimate body composition is by the use of special calipers that essentially *pinch* people at different parts of the body. This method is made possible because a relationship exists between the fat just under the skin and one's total amount of body fat.[27] The caliper device measures the thickness of various skinfolds. This information is plugged into equations to calculate an estimation of body composition. When performed correctly, the skin fold technique may be accurate to about ± 3%. Various equations exist for skinfold analysis of body composition, with each using different sites that can be pinched. When using skinfold analysis make sure that the equation you are using corresponds to the sites you are pinching. For example, there is an equation specific to testing only three sites. Fitness professionals must make sure also that they measure the sites specified by the equation. Measuring the wrong sites reduces accuracy. Also, skin fold measurements are always taken on the right side of the body only. While research shows that when done properly, skin fold analysis can provide relatively good estimates of body composition, some drawbacks to this technique include:

1. Total body fat does not just depend on the fat under the skin. Skin fold analysis cannot determine fat around organs.

2. The degree of accuracy of skin fold analysis depends on the expertise of the person performing the test.

3. Equations for this method are gender, age and race specific. Thus, using the wrong equation will generate a less accurate result.

4. Some people are not comfortable being pinched by people they do not know.

5. This method may not be appropriate for the very obese

Bioelectric Impedance Analysis

Bioelectric impedance analysis (BIA) represents an easy to administer technique for assessing body composition, which makes it very popular in fitness and wellness centers. Bioelectric impedance analysis works by passing a low intensity electric current through the body and measuring its resistance.[2] Because fat is not a good conductor of electricity, the greater the fat mass a person has, the greater the resistance and hence, the slower the current passes through the body. In this way, BIA is able to provide a quick and relatively accurate estimate of body composition. BIA devices usually cost about $50 and come in hand-held versions and those that a person can stand on. In addition to estimating percent body fat, some models may also calculate BMI as well. Some models may also have an "athlete mode" which may provide a greater degree of accuracy for those who exercise on a regular basis. Whichever type is chosen, the accuracy of BIA, depends on several guidelines:

General BIA Guidelines

1. Do not eat or drink for at least four hours before the test
2. Do not exercise at least 12 hours before the test
3. Do urinate 30 minutes before the test
4. Do not drink alcohol at least 48 hours before the test
5. Do not ingest any diuretics (including caffeine) before the test unless prescribed by a physician

In addition, another factor to consider with BIA is the equation being used to determine body composition.[2] Many BIA equations exist. The equations used today in commercially available machines are probably good for most individuals however, some machines may be unable to determine body composition on those falling outside what the machine *thinks* is normal. Circumstances where the machine may be unable to determine body compassion include people over 300 pounds as well as bodybuilders and other professional athletes who have unusually low body fat percentages.

One group where BIA should not be used are in those who have pacemakers, defibrillators or other implantable heart devices. The electrical signal may accidentally activate these machines. Fitness professionals should ask everyone, regardless of age, as to whether they have a pacemaker, defibrillator or similar device. Likewise, BIA should not be performed on pregnant women.

Near Infrared Interactance

The estimation of body composition by near infrared interactance (NIR) makes use of a specialized probe that is placed against an area of the body (e.g. the biceps) which emits infrared light that is passed through muscle and fat. Fat and muscle will absorb different frequencies of light. The difference between them is entered into prediction equations along with information on age, height, weight and activity level to estimate body composition. While variations of this technique have been used in clinical settings since the 1960s, portable devices that are commercially available have been shown to be less accurate than skin fold techniques and bioelectric impedance analysis, described above. Some research hints that NIR may be less accurate in those who exercise.[123] Other research finds that NIR might overestimate body fatness in lean people and underestimate it in overweight people. More study is needed before NIR is universally accepted.

Hydrostatic Weighing

Hydrostatic weighing is often called the "gold standard" of body composition analysis because it is the most accurate method and the basis upon which all the others are compared. Because of this, hydrostatic weighing is often used in clinical research. The other name for this technique is *underwater weighing*, a phrase derived from the fact that individuals are completely submerged in water to determine body composition.

Hydrostatic weighing is based on *Archimedes's Principle*—that is, a body buoyed in water will be forced to the surface by a force equal to the volume of water that it displaces. Stating this another way, fat floats; the more fat a person has on their body, the lighter they will be when weighted under the water. When having body composition determined by this method, the person usually sits on a specialized scale and is completely submerged in water. The individual then forcibly exhales as much air out of their lungs as possible and remains motionless. For individuals who are uncomfortable with being submerged under the water as well as those who are not comfortable being in a bathing suit, this method can be a frightening experience. Because special equipment is required, underwater weighing is more likely to be offered at a university that has a physical education department as opposed to a health club setting.

Air Displacement

Just as hydrostatic weighing measures the displacement of water, body composition can also be determined by measuring the amount of air that a person displaces. The most popular of these types of machines is the Bod Pod®, which measures air displacement when people sit in a special chamber. Clinical studies have been published on the Bod Pod and some find it to be almost as accurate as hydrostatic weighing in a variety of populations.[34,53] While body composition can be determined in a matter of minutes, one possible drawback is the price, which can be tens of thousands of dollars. In addition, not all studies have found air displacement to be as accurate as hydrostatic weighing for all individuals.[33,55,56] Thus, more research is warranted on air displacement before is universally accepted for all populations.

Dual Energy X-Ray Absorptiometry

In addition to its more common use—determining bone density—dual energy x-ray absorptiometry (or *DEXA Scan* as its also called) can also very precisely estimate the amount of fat and lean muscle tissue that is present. Like the Bod Pod®, described previously, DEXA is quite expensive. More importantly than the price, because it uses low level radiation, DEXA is very unlikely to be found at any health club but rather is reserved for hospitals and other clinical research settings.

Chapter 11

Diets and Weight Loss

Americans spend over 30 billion dollars a year on a myriad of books, potions, pills, and exercise devices touted to aid in shedding excess bodyweight.[38] The reality however is that 95% of any weight that is lost by these methods is probably regained eventually. Another sad reality is that the vast majority of diets don't appear to work long-term for all people. This makes the job of the fitness professional who espouses the time tested concepts of *calories in, calories out*, to be especially difficult. In reality however, this actually is the premise of many popular diets on the lips of people today. In other words, most diets get people to reduce the number of calories they eat. This chapter will deal with many of the most popular diets on the market today. The goals for this chapter are to arm the fitness professional with the knowledge to help their clients safely navigate though the hype and sometimes odd approaches which seem to be all too common in the world of weight loss.

Low Carb Diets

By far, one of the most popular diets in recent history has been the low carbohydrate diet. Low carb diets are sometimes called ketogenic diets because they tend to produce acid-like molecules called ketones.

People usually report losing a significant amount of weight during the first few weeks of a low carbohydrate diet. There is actually a very good reason for this. All humans store excess carbohydrates in the form of glycogen. When carbohydrates are not eaten or when their intake is severely curtailed, the body slowly starts to break down its stored glycogen reserves to maintain blood sugar levels. As glycogen is degraded to glucose, a lot of water is also released in the process. In fact, every gram of glycogen liberates about 3 grams of water. This is why one of the first things people notice on a low carb diet is the almost constant urge to go to urinate. After a week or two, a significant amount of weight is lost, however most of it is in the form of water. Low carb diets can be rather difficult to maintain long-term because carbohydrates are our body's preferred fuel source. This lack of carbs can lead to fatigue and a decrease in aerobic exercise capacity. While the long-term safety of low carb diets on cardiovascular health is still not known, studies to date generally find them safe for short-term usage. Research however also hints that long term use may not be more effective than simply eating less. In one of the longest studies of this diet to date, 63 overweight individuals were followed for one year.[124] About half of the individuals followed the Atkins diet while the other half, ate a lower calorie diet (1200-1800 calories per day) where the majority of calories (60%) came from carbohydrates. For the first 6 months, the Atkins group lost about 4% more weight than the calorie counting group. However, after one year, there was no significant difference in the amount of weight lost by either group. A longer study was published in the New England Journal of Medicine in 2008).[132] This study lasted two years and found that an Atkins-type diet (where 40% of calories came from fat) resulted in more weight loss than a low fat or Mediterranean-type diet which used 30% and 33% fat respectively. The average weight loss for the low carb group was 10.3 pounds over the two year course of the study. The low fat and Mediterranean groups lost 6.3 and 9.7 pounds respectively. Thus, the difference in weight lost between the groups was not much. In addition, considering the two year duration of the study, relatively little weight was lost across the board. All groups were highly monitored by researchers and the low carb group was advised to keep low their intake of saturated and trans fats. This, either alone or in combination with the weight loss, may have resulted in the favorable effects on the cholesterol/HDL ratio noticed in the low carb group.

High Protein Diets

High protein diets necessitate that individuals consume larger amounts of dietary protein, often in excess of the RDA (0.8 g/kg BW). Proponents of high protein diets claim that elevated protein intakes may lead to weight loss because protein may temporarily suppress the appetite and force the body to rely on fat as a fuel source.[36] A more logical reason however is related to water loss associated with glycogen depletion. Very high protein diets (several times the RDA) may also be accompanied by such unwanted side effects as electrolyte imbalances and altered pH levels via ketone accumulation.[45] On the plus side, issues of kidney problems resulting from high protein diets appear to be less of a issue than once thought.[72] Protein does tend to slow digestion and also seems to raise metabolism more than carbohydrate or fat. Another mechanism that may be responsible for the weight loss observed on these diets is that protein doesn't have a lot of calories (only 4 calories per gram). While a slightly higher level of protein may help some people reduce weight, a problem arises when protein is consumed at the expense of other healthy foods that the body also needs. People who advocate high protein diets usually forget that all food is health food, when used in moderation. High intakes of protein are not advised for people with kidney or liver disease because it may make their condition worse.

Low Fat Diets

Before low carbohydrate diets, there were low fat diets. At the heart of many low fat diets is a reduction in calories. Thus, many low fat diets are low calorie diets. Each gram of fat has 9 calories –more than either protein or carbohydrate (which each have about 4 calories per gram). So when people begin cutting fat out of their diet (or cutting fat grams as some diets advocate), they are really cutting back on a lot of calories. These types of diets also tend to place an emphasis on fruits and vegetables which, are also low in calories. From a health perspective, a low fat, high fruit and vegetable diet may be beneficial because high fat diets have been linked to diseases like some cancers and heart disease. Low fat diets that also emphasize fruits and vegetables may compliment each other by nature of the phytonutrient content of these foods which emerging evidence hints may also reduce disease risk. However, the bottom line is that while from a health standpoint, low fat diets may be advantageous, from a weight loss standpoint, most are just low in calories.

Of all the low fat diets, one in particular stands out. It is called the Ornish Diet, named after Dean Ornish a medical doctor and researcher. The Ornish diet consists of a very low fat diet (about 10% of total calories coming from fat), daily aerobic exercise and stress reduction techniques like meditation. Research has been conducted on the Ornish diet and published in peer-reviewed medical journals finding it can produce weight loss.[125] However the real reason people may be interested in the Ornish diet has to do with reversal of the buildup of artery clogging plaque. Research on the Ornish diet has noted significant reductions in plaque buildup after sticking with the diet for up to a year. Research notes that the Ornish diet may lower LDL (bad cholesterol) as well as C-reactive protein (CRP) which is also implicated in heart disease development. The Ornish diet also places an emphasis on daily, moderate intensity aerobic exercise to help boost HDL and burn calories. Because stress can also contribute to heart disease, another aspect of the Ornish plan is its emphasis of stress reduction techniques like yoga and mediation and social support.

Acid/Alkaline Diets

Alkaline good, acid bad. This is the premise of diets that theorize that when our bodies become too acid (by eating the wrong types of foods) that weight gain and disease develops. When delving into these types of diets, readers quickly encounter the term "pH" so let's define it here. pH is a chemistry term that refers to the degree of acidity, which in turn is related to the amount of hydrogen atoms present (this is where the *H* in pH comes from). The pH scale is from 0 to 14 where a rating of 0 is very acid and a pH of 14 is very alkaline (also called basic). Another way of describing this is to define an acid as anything that releases hydrogen into a system. Something that is alkaline removes hydrogen atoms. According the Environmental Protection Agency, sulfuric acid has a pH of 1 while pure water has a pH of 8. Bleach is very alkaline with a pH of 13. Human blood has a pH of about 7.35 -7.4. So, human blood tends to be a little on the alkaline side. That being said, human blood has a very narrow range of pH at which life can be sustained. Thus, the body usually does everything it can to maintain its blood at its normal pH. In fact, if we couldn't buffer against large increases in blood acidity (or alkalinity), drinking a glass of orange juice (pH of 3.5) would surely kill us! More specifically stated, a blood pH as low as 6.8 or as high as 8.0 is deadly.[126] Because of the body's desire to maintain a blood pH of about 7.35 - 7.4 and the disastrous consequences of not being able to, the questions then become:

1. Is it possible to significantly alter the pH of the body for any length of time?
2. Does long term altered pH cause chronic disease and weight gain?

Unfortunately the answers to both of these questions is not well known. Currently pH based diets have not undergone scientific scrutiny. Outside of diet books, evidence in support of these regimens have not yet been published in peer-reviewed nutrition or medical journals and many scientists are skeptical of their claims. All this doesn't necessarily mean these diets won't work but rather that there is no conclusive proof as of yet.

Sometimes people wanting to know the pH of the body will test their saliva or urine. The problem with doing this is that saliva and urine pH may not be the same as the pH inside the body. As a result, testing these fluids may not be reliable indicators.

Foods said to be alkaline include most fruits and vegetables. Thus, a general guideline for those who want to alkalize their diet includes eating more fruits and vegetables, which as mentioned previously are low in calories. By adding these foods to the diet and eliminating supposed acid producing foods like chocolate, salad dressing, peanuts, soft drinks and sugary breakfast cereals, probably would reduce weight. But, is the weight that's lost due to eating fewer calories or because of the acid/alkaline balance of the diet?

Cabbage Soup Diet

The cabbage soup diet has been around for decades and many people still believe that there is something magical about this method although in reality nothing can be farther from the truth. How many calories are in cabbage soup? Not many. By eating only cabbage soup or mostly cabbage soup, people cut back on a large number of calories which in turn signals the body to begin breaking down its glycogen reserves. As mentioned previously, this releases a large volume of water into the circulation, resulting in frequent trips to the bathroom. So, while the cabbage soup diet, might promote short-term water weight loss, in the long run, it's difficult to stick to because its boring and humans need more than cabbage soup to survive and thrive. The cabbage soup diet is one of many one-food-centered diets that that abound on the internet. Another classic variation is the grapefruit diet. It too is a low calorie diet.

Blood Type-Based Diets

Blood type-based diets advocate that a person's blood type determines what foods he or she should eat. Eating right for your blood type, say advocates, can help reduce weight as well as improve overall health. For example, a person with type A blood might avoid meats and predominately eat vegetables. A person with type O blood should eat a high protein, low carbohydrate diet. The problem with blood type diets is that they have not been rigorously tested scientifically to see if there is something to them or not.

Food Combining Diets

Some diet books are based on the notion that humans cannot adequately digest and absorb certain combinations of foods when they are eaten in the same meal. For example, some variations may state that carbohydrates should not be eaten with meats or that people should not eat fruit and meat at the same meal. According to these diets, weight loss and health results when the *correct* combinations of foods are eaten. Unfortunately, the bulk of the published, peer-reviewed nutrition and medical literature does not support the theory that we can only absorb certain combinations of foods or that only certain groupings of foods promotes weight loss. Some variations of this diet regimen call for eating only fruits or only vegetables for the first week or two. Because fruits and vegetables tend to be low in calories, this might be the reason people lose weight with this type of diet.

Zone-Type Diets

Some diets advocate that weight loss can only occur when people eat carbohydrates, proteins and fats in specific percentages. While several variations of this concept exist, the most popular over the last decade has been the *Zone Diet* which advocates that weight loss and improved health are found by striving to have each meal be composed of 40% carbohydrate, 30% protein and 30% fat. It is said that eating foods in these specific combinations puts one in the "zone". At the heart of many of these diets is the claim eating foods in the 40, 30, 30 combination will better stabilize insulin levels. According to advocates, insulin, while a vital hormone, is responsible for obesity and various diseases. While the carbohydrate amount specified in these diets (40%) is less than that advocated by many nutrition educators, these diets are overall pretty healthy. Most diets emphasize fruits, vegetables, lean meats and low fat products and restricts indulgence in foods that contain saturated fats. Some have criticized these diets because they tend to be relatively low in calcium and whole grains.[127] One drawback to the Zone-type diets is that they may be difficult to precisely calculate the proportions specified; however, because they do not totally eliminate any one food group, people may find it easier to stick with them. The fact that the zone diet emphasizes fruits and vegetables at every meal probably means it is low in calories. Some research has been conducted on the Zone diet and found it can help reduce weight.[125] Whether this effect is due to the diet decreasing insulin levels or because it's a low calorie diet, requires further research.

Raw Food Diets

Advocates of raw food-type diets feel that most—if not all—cooked foods are bad for us and that health and weight loss are best achieved when eating food in its natural state (raw). According to raw food diet theory, by not cooking foods, one preserves enzymes and other vital nutrients that help keep us healthy. Raw food-based diets tend to be filled with nutrient-dense fruits and vegetables and low in calories. This reduction in calorie content is probably the reason why the diet reduces weight. Raw food diets also tend to emphasize organically grown foods which contain far less chemicals, hormones, pesticides and antibiotics. These diets are also usually low in fat (especially saturated fat) and have a higher fiber content, which helps slow digestion, making people feel fuller longer. On the other hand, some nutrients like lycopene and beta carotene for example are more bioavailable after cooking. In theory, some variations of raw food diets may be deficient in nutrients like vitamin B-12 and calcium. Eating foods in their raw state may make it difficult for some with digestion problems as well. Overall diets based on raw foods, are pretty healthy and most likely will result in weight loss because of their emphasis in nutrient-dense, low calorie fruits and vegetables. Diets of this type might also reduce the risk of several diseases like cancer, diabetes and heart disease. Depending on how *back to basics* a person gets with raw food type diets, a good multivitamin as well as a calcium supplement might also be something to consider.

Body For Life®

The Body For Life® program was developed by the makers of EAS line of dietary supplements and popularized by the book *Body For Life* by Bill Philips. One of the advantages of this program is that it's less of a diet than a lifestyle change plan. The program emphasizes eating about 6 meals a day with each meal made up of about 300 calories (so, about 1800 calories a day are eaten). This is less than many people already eat so this program would probably promote weight loss. Each meal should also contain some lean protein like chicken or fish to help raise metabolism and promote muscle growth.

In addition, the Body For Life program does something that most other diets don't do and that's place a big emphasis on exercise–specifically strength training. In a nutshell, the program advocates a pyramid-up system of strength training whereby a person lifts a weight for 12 reps, followed by a set for 10 reps and then 8 reps and then a set for 6 reps. Approximately 30 seconds to 1 minute rest periods are taken between sets. Cardiovascular exercise is limited to about 20 minutes at a high intensity. Needless to say, this is a very aggressive strength training program and beginners might want to do at least a month of strength training at lower intensities to prepare for it. One of the most interesting aspects of Body For Life is its emphasis on making smart food choices and trying to get readers to determine why they make bad choices. This might make this program more well rounded than other diets.

Diet Program	Emphasis	How it Works / Notes
Atkins Diet	Reduce carbohydrates	Glycogen/water loss in beginning. Possible consumption of less calories long-term.
High Protein Diets	Higher protein intakes	Glycogen/water loss in beginning. Protein may boost metabolism and slow digestion.
Low Fat Diets	Reduce fat consumption	Reducing fat, really reduces calories. Low fat diets may reduce disease risk.
Acid/Alkaline Diets	Eat more alkaline foods like fruits and vegetables	Fruits and vegetables are low in calories. Diet's impact on disease reduction is unknown.
Cabbage Soup diet	Eat cabbage soup	Cabbage soup is low in calories. Promotes glycogen and water loss.

Diet Program	Emphasis	How it Works / Notes
Grapefruit Diet	Eat grapefruit	Grapefruit is low in calories. Promotes glycogen and water loss. Grapefruit not appropriate for people using some medications
Blood Type-Based Diets	Eat foods according to your blood type	No published peer-reviewed evidence to support diets claims.
Food Combining Diets	Eat only specific combinations of foods	No published peer-reviewed evidence to support diets claims.
Zone-Type Diets	Eat Fruits, vegetables, lean meats in 40% 30% 30% combination	Diet is low in calories
Raw Food Diets	Eat only or mostly foods in their raw state	Diet is low in calories
Body For Life Diet	Eat several small means during the day plus regular exercise.	Low calories plus exercise promotes weight loss/gain in muscle.
Ornish Diet	Eat a very low fat diet plus daily aerobic exercise & stress reduction	Diet is low in calories. Only diet to date clinically shown to reverse artery clogging plaque.

Questions to Ask About Diets

The following are a series of questions to ask when researching a diet:

1. How is the diet different from all the others out there?
2. Is the diet a low calorie diet?
3. Is there any published on the diet that clinically proves it works?
4. Does the diet program recommend or advocate questionable dietary supplements to help "support" weight loss? If yes, ask for published peer-reviewed research that proves the products work.
5. Does the diet program advocate restricting any single food group? If yes, this is probably unhealthy.
6. Is the diet something people can easily fit into their lifestyle for the long run?.

Fitness professionals should remember that most diets will probably work in the short term. The fact however that the majority of dieters fail means that most have a miserable long-term track record. Diets are a short-term fix and nothing more. One of the toughest challenges that face fitness professionals today is helping people realize that real change comes not with the latest fad diet but from recognizing the lifestyle habits that brought them to where they are now, and taking reasonable and attainable steps to a more healthy way of life.

Chapter 12

Supermarket Self Defense

Health and fitness guru, Jack La Lanne, once remarked that *dying is easy, staying alive is the hard part*. Jack was right! Staying healthy is 24/7 job to be to sure. For some, working out may be the easy part because that takes a tangible effort on their part. The more difficult area for people may be the eating part and for many, there is no greater stress to overindulge than when at their local supermarket. This makes perfect sense. Think about it; everything is right there at you fingertips, just waiting to be seen and eaten! Believe it or not, supermarkets are actually designed this way! Whether you know it or not, everything in the supermarket is specifically arranged so that you will spend the maximum amount of time shopping. The longer your stay in the supermarket, the more money you will probably spend. Because there is a method to this madness, let's go over some of the design tactics used by today's big supermarket chains—as well as the local mom and pop stores in your neighborhood—and see how they get you to buy things you might not ordinarily buy.

Did you ever notice that whenever you enter a supermarket, you almost always have to walk through the fruit and vegetable section before you can get to the stuff you want? It's no accident that this happens. Supermarket owners know (because they hire experts who do research on this) that the arrangement and aroma of all those fruits and vegetables has a big effect on people in terms of what they buy. An interesting little tid bit about the produce section of supermarkets is that it may generate almost 20 percent of the supermarkets profits while only taking up about 10 percent of the store's space! The produce section is usually the second most profitable area in the typical supermarket. It's also not an accident that the veggies are found along the walls of most supermarkets. This is because a sizable amount of profits for the supermarket are generated by products that are aligned along the walls. So the more time you spend hunting along the perimeter of the supermarket, the more money you are likely to spend.

If the produce section is the second most lucrative section in the supermarket, what do you think is the # 1 ticket item? It's the meat section. Everybody (except maybe vegetarians) eats meat at least once in a while so it makes perfect sense that this would be the area where supermarkets would generate the most revenue. The meat section is also strategically placed—usually along the back wall of the supermarket. The meat section is placed here so you're most likely to run into it whenever you exit from an isle. You exit an aisle and poof - there it is! And people, being the *Pavlovian* dogs that we are, say to ourselves *you know, I would really like to have hot-dogs for dinner tonight*!

What about the dairy section? It's usually placed as far from the entrance as possible. The reason for this is that everybody usually buys milk or eggs when they go food shopping. Therefore, it's in the supermarket's best interest to *lead* you through as much of its gauntlet of goodies as possible before you get to the dairy section. In addition, when you finally do arrive at the dairy section, you'll find that popular items like milk, are usually placed at one end of the dairy display and stuff like butter is usually at the other end. This way, the supermarket gets you to look at all the other, less popular stuff in between.

Another way supermarkets try to get you to buy stuff is with the width of the shopping carts. Sometimes the carts are so wide that it's hard to move through the narrow aisles of the supermarket. This is especially true if there are others in the aisle with you. The slower you move, the more likely you are to see something and buy it. Some have estimated that for every unplanned extra minute we spend in the supermarket, that we spend an extra $2.

What about those free samples that we are sometimes offered while shopping? Are they really free? Not really if you decide to by the product. Free samples are another way supermarkets entice us to buy what we ordinarily wouldn't.

When you're in the checkout line, you're basically a captive audience with no place to go. So, while you are standing there, waiting patiently they hit you again with stuff that you might not ordinarily buy. Take a close look at those areas the next time you're at the market. What you'll usually find is an assortment of candy, magazines, batteries, and even little toys. The toys and candy are strategically placed low to the ground, where small children can see them. Because adults are more likely to think about their breath, breath mints and similar items are placed higher up, closer to adult eye level. Some supermarkets even have TV displays that advertise products when you're waiting in line.

What about those "preferred customer cards" that all supermarkets give out these days? While these cards do offer some discounts to those who present them at checkout, they are really designed to track the items you buy and send you coupons to get you to buy more stuff.

The best way for people to protect themselves is to create a shopping list before going to the supermarket. Knowing a head of time what you are going to buy will go a long way at reducing the time you spend wandering aimlessly past the thousands of items which clamor for your attention.

Another way to protect yourself from buying items you ordinarily would not purchase is to never go to the supermarket on an empty stomach. We are much more susceptible to the enticements of cookies, cakes and other edible goodies when we arrive at the supermarket hungry.

The Big Picture

Deceptive as all of this may seem, in reality, it's really just capitalism and supermarkets are not the only ones who do this. Supermarkets sell food just the same way as vitamin stores sell vitamins, car dealerships sell cars, health clubs sell fitness and personal trainers sell health, fitness, knowledge and hope. The goal in this chapter is not to make you believe that there is a vast conspiracy to get people to eat but rather to alert fitness professionals to these facts so that they can better help people make wiser food choices. Some fitness professionals may want to go to the supermarket with their clients to help educate them further. For those who do this on a regular basis, it's probably wise to contact the supermarket ahead of time to make sure its ok. Some supermarkets that cater to health conscious people may even welcome the addition of a certified fitness professional and use him/her as a selling point. The bottom line is that in moderation, all food is basically health food. Helping people recognize this fact and avoid the pitfalls of too much overindulging is a laudable service that all fitness professionals should practice with their clients.

Chapter 13

Exercise & Weight Control

Exercise is an integral component of any sound weight loss program. Exercise burns calories and as such, is one of the best ways people can use to promote weight loss. Studies of the National Weight Control Registry, a database of people who were successful at long-term (i.e., greater than one year) weight loss, show that exercise was an important component of weight loss success. While many opt for aerobic exercise training when losing weight, resistance strength training can help also given that every pound of extra muscle is estimated consume an extra 30-50 calories per day.[41] Thus, in theory, the greater the amount of lean muscle tissue one has, the greater the amount of overall calories burned in a given time period. This, in turn, may lead to greater weight loss in the long run. In addition, evidence suggests that combining exercise with a reduced calorie intake enhances the amount of weight that is lost as fat.[9] Individuals most successful at losing weight and preventing the regaining of weight often report exercising at least 280 minutes per week.[1] This amounts to:

- 40 minutes a day if working out 7 days a week

- 56 minutes a day if working out 5 days a week

- 70 minutes a day if working out 4 days a week

- 93 minutes a day if working out 3 days a week

Notice that the numbers above are greater than the often quoted 30 minutes per day, 3-5 days per week for general cardiovascular health. Because not everybody can commit to large amounts of exercise on a daily basis, it's important to combine exercise with mild calorie restriction. Exercise alone, is unlikely to cause significant weight loss in most people.

Types of Exercise

When deciding on an exercise program, people basically have two broad categories of choices: aerobic exercise and anaerobic exercise (strength training). Both types of exercise offer advantages for the person looking to improve health, quality of life and weight loss. As a rule aerobic exercise tends to burn a lot of calories during the activity. Generally, when prescribing aerobic exercise, individuals should chose activities that incorporate the large muscles of the body such as the legs, chest and back. These types of exercise have a higher metabolic cost associated with them (in other words, they burn more calories). Health club machines that are appropriate for this include treadmills, steppers, elliptical machines and rowers to name a few. For those not used to a regular exercise program, performing the activity 2 to 3 days a week and building up to 4 to 5 days a week is usually advocated. When designing an exercise program for a beginner, fitness professionals should place a greater emphasis on the *duration* of exercise rather than *intensity* of exercise. This is because greater exercise intensity is associated with greater risk of injury.

At the other end of the exercise spectrum is anaerobic exercise like strength training. Strength training, while generally burning a little fewer calories than aerobic exercise, improves muscle strength and may elevate metabolic rate for longer periods of time after the activity ceases. Thus, strength training may help people burn more calories when they are sleeping! Like aerobic exercise mentioned previously, the emphasis here should also should be on the large muscle groups of the body to maximize calorie utilization. People will burn more calories doing a chest press than biceps curls, for example. Because many overweight individuals may not be accustomed to exercise, starting with one set of 10-15 repetitions for the major muscle groups of the body (chest, back, legs) will be easier and less likely to result in delayed onset muscle soreness (DOMS), a possible hindrance to continuation of exercise. Generally, strength training should be performed two to three days a week.

When dealing with those new to exercise, fitness professionals should be aware that exercise drop-out rates increase when workouts last longer than 60 minutes. Because of this, circuit training might be ideal for new exercisers and those trying to lose weight because it offers a variety of exercises in a short period of time, is not perceived as boring and places less stress on muscles and joints. Many fitness professionals are enthusiastic about their profession and want everybody to be as passionate about health and wellness as they are. For some people, *Rome was not built in a day* and small steps may be needed. Showing people how they can incorporate an effective exercise program into a busy lifestyle can go a long way to keeping a client motivated and on the road to better health for years to come.

Exercise Intensity vs. Exercise Duration

Exercise duration refers to the time spent working out during an exercise session. Exercise intensity refers to how hard or intense the workout feels. Studies show that at lower intensities of exercise, people tend to burn greater percentages of fat than at higher intensities. This has led some to believe that lower intensities of exercise are always best for fat loss. In fact some treadmills, ellipticals and bikes actually have a "fat burn" program that is based on this notion. On the other hand, higher intensities of exercise are associated with greater calories being used. So which is the best option to use? It turns out that both of points of view have merit. When deciding which is appropriate for the client—higher intensity or longer duration—the fitness professional should always consider the initial fitness of the client. Individuals who are not accustomed to physical exertion are best served by lower intensity activity or in the case of the very deconditioned, even intermittent activity. This will allow the deconditioned individual to exercise for a longer period of time and thus result in a greater amount of calories being consumed. A general rule of thumb for the fitness professional should be to increase the time (duration) of activity before increasing the intensity of activity. After the individual can successfully achieve 20-60 minutes of low to moderate level activity with no discomfort, fitness professionals may wish to adjust the intensity of the activity to further stimulate metabolic changes.

Measuring Exercise Intensity

Exercise intensity can be measured by a variety of techniques. Not all techniques are appropriate for all people. The fitness professional must be aware of the variety of ways to measure exercise intensity and those that are best suited for their clients. The most common techniques are listed below:

The Talk Test

The talk test is one of the simplest ways to gauge exercise intensity. The fitness professional essentially talks to the client while he/she is working out—and lets the client do most of the talking. If the client can talk without undue difficulty, then exercise may be deemed well tolerated. If the client has trouble talking or cannot talk during exercise, then the intensity should be reduced to where they can talk. This method works very well for people performing aerobic exercise and circuit training and because it requires no math or special equipment can be done *on the fly*. As such, it's popular in exercise classes.

Percent of Maximum Heart Rate

It is not uncommon for fitness professionals to prescribe a target heart rate (THR) training zone for exercise and to have clients exercise within this zone. The easiest way to assign this training zone is by first determining the client's estimated maximal number of heart beats per min (also called *estimated maximal heart rate*) and then take percentages of this number. The determination of estimated maximum heart rate is usually achieved by the equation "220 – Age". For example, if an individual was 20 years old, he or she would have an estimated maximum heart rate of 220 – 20 = 200 heart beats per minute. This means that theoretically, the heart of a 20 year old individual will beat no more than about 200 times in one minute. Now that the estimated maximum heart rate is known, percentages of this number can be calculated. Let's continue the example above and suppose that the fitness professional wanted to calculate 60% and 75% of estimated maximal heart rate:

$$200 \times 0.60 = 120 \text{ bpm}$$

$$200 \times 0.75 = 150 \text{ bpm}$$

So according to this example, the person would exercise at a heart rate of between 120 and 150 heart beats per min (often abbreviated as bpm). This corresponds to 60% and 75% of the person's estimated maximal ability. Any percent the fitness professional is looking to achieve can be estimated with this simple equation. For safety reasons, it is probably wise to start at lower percentages such as 50-65% when first working with a new client to get a better idea of how much exercise they can tolerate.

This is also important because the calculation of maximal heart rate is an *estimate* and thus, is not completely accurate. In fact, calculation of maximal heart rate from the *220 minus Age* equation may underestimate one's true maximal heart rate.

Karvonen Heart Rate Formula

Because the 220-Age formula described previously is not 100% accurate, some fitness professionals opt to calculate target heart rate training zones by another method called the *Karvonen Heart Rate Formula*. This method is usually seen as more accurate than simply taking percentages of estimated maximum heart rate. To use the Karvonen formula, the resting heart rate and age of the individual must be known. The fitness professional can either measure resting heart rate him or herself after having the client rest quietly for several minutes, or they can teach their client's to measure resting heart rate themselves, preferably in the morning just after waking. The steps of the Karvonen formula are as follows:

Step 1: 220 - age

Step 2: subtract resting heart rate from step 1

Step 3: multiply result of step 2 by percentages you wish to calculate

Step 4: add resting heart rate to results of step 3

Just as before, let's demonstrate the Karvonen method with an example.
Subject: a 30 year old female with a resting heart rate of 60 beats per min. The fitness professional wants to calculate 60% and 80% using the Karvonen method.

Step 1: 220 – 30 = 190 bpm

Step 2: 190 – 60 = 130 bpm

Step 3: 130 X 0.6 = 78 & 130 X 0.8 = 104

Step 4: 78 + 60 = **138** & 104 + 60 = **164**

Answer: Target heart rate is 138 to 164 beats per minute

The ACSM generally recommends 60% and 80% when calculating target heart rate ranges for apparently healthy individuals.[1] In reality however, fitness professionals can calculate any percentages in light of the fact that some people (frail, elderly, deconditioned, etc.) may not be able to exercise aerobically at 60 to 80% Karvonen heart rate maximum for prolonged periods of time. When in doubt, being conservative with new clients is ok.

Ratings of Perceived Exertion

Ratings of perceived exertion (or RPE) is essentially a zero to 10 scale whereby a person rates how intense they perceive their exercise exertion level to be. The other name for this method is Borg Scale.

RPE Scale

Rating	Meaning
0	Nothing at all
1	Very weak effort
2	Weak effort
3	Moderately strong or difficult effort
5	Strong or difficult effort
7	Very strong or difficult effort
10	Maximal effort

Where the numbers are not in perfect order (for example, between 5 and 7) it is understood that the number that is missing would be a level of intensity in-between. For example, in the table above, level 6 is missing between level 5 and level 7. This indicates that level 6 is an exercise intensity between level 5 and 7.

The RPE scale is very flexible and can be used to gauge difficulty during aerobic exercise (*how difficult is this level feel on a scale from zero to 10?*) and strength training (*how heavy does that weight feel on a zero to 10 scale?*). Some even use RPE to determine fatigue level (*how fatigued do you feel on scale from zero to 10?*). The RPE scale is also an accepted method for gauging exercise intensity in people with high blood pressure who are on medications that lower resting heart rate. One draw back to the RPE scale is that people must be familiar with what the numbers mean. In other words, asking somebody how they feel on a zero to 10 scale won't produce an accurate result if the client has no idea what the numbers mean.

Volume of Oxygen

One of the most commonly used clinical measurements of aerobic fitness is the maximum volume of oxygen test often abbreviated as VO_{2max} It is called "VO_2" because the letter V stands for *volume* and O_2 is the chemical symbol for *oxygen*. The VO_2 test is a measure of how efficient we are at making energy (ATP) aerobically. As exercise intensity increases, we tend to breathe harder, taking in more oxygen which results in an increase in VO_2. At some point during the VO_2 test however, VO_2 will not increase as the exercise demand increases. Now, the individual is said to have reached VO_{2max} which is the maximum volume of oxygen that can be consumed by the body to make energy aerobically. When a person is exercising at their VO_{2max} they are essentially working as hard as they can.

Most healthy individuals will have a VO_{2max} of between 30-40 milliliters of oxygen per kilogram of body weight per minute, This is usually abbreviated as 30 to 40 ml O_2 /kg BW/min. A kilogram is equal to 2.2 pounds. If we were to break a person down into kilogram increments, this means that on average, most people would only use between 30 to 40 milliliters of oxygen per kilogram of their body their weight per minute, when pushed to their absolute maximum. The VO_{2max} of aerobically-trained athletes tends to be higher and is generally over 50 milliliters of oxygen per kilogram of body weight per minute. While VO_{2max} does have a genetic component, exercise training can result in a greater VO_{2max} being achieved. The determination of VO_{2max} is usually not measured in a fitness center setting. Because of the risks associated with pushing people to their absolute limit, VO_{2max} is often calculated in the presence of a physician or other qualified exercise scientist and requires the use of expensive equipment. Some pieces of equipment in health clubs today however may make it possible to estimate the VO_2 that a person is exercising at. This brings us to the next topic, called METs.

Metabolic Equivalents

The term METs stands for Metabolic Equivalents. This method is based upon the fact that at rest, every kilogram (2.2 lb.) of body weight burns 3.5 milliliters of oxygen per minute. This value of 3.5 milliliters of oxygen per kilogram of body weight per minute is referred to as 1 MET. This means that at rest, every 2.2 pound segment of your body (that is, every kilogram of your body weight) consumes exactly 3.5 milliliters of oxygen per minute. Because of this, the intensity of activity can be described in terms of METs. For example, an activity that is 2 METs is twice as intense as resting. An activity that is 5 METs is five times as intense as that experienced at rest. This also means that the higher the MET level, the greater the calories consumed. Other ways to define METs include:

- 1MET = basal metabolic rate (BMR)
- 1MET=resting VO_2

Because 1MET can also be referred to as resting VO_2 and because 1 MET is equal to 3.5 ml O_2 / Kg BW/Min means that the number 3.5 can be used to convert METs to VO_2 and vice versa. For example, suppose someone is exercising on a treadmill at an intensity of 15 METs. Their VO_2 at that level is 15 X 3.5 = 52.5 ml O_2 / Kg BW/min. Thus, METs and VO_2 are almost the same thing, just stated in different languages. Many common exercise machines in health clubs today provide estimations of METs. METs is also a common way in which medical professionals define exercise intensity. For more information on exercise, read my book *Personal Fitness Training: Beyond the Basics*, available at my website www.Joe-Cannon.com

116

Chapter 14

How to Read a Food Label

A central theme that runs silently through all of the topics relevant to the fitness professional is that of an educator. In fact, it has been the experience of this author that one of the main reasons people seek the guidance of a fitness professional is due their desire to gain knowledge on health, wellness and fitness-related topics. To some individuals, one of the biggest mysteries in nutrition today sits quietly in every kitchen cabinet in America—the food label. This chapter will present an overview of the major parts of the food label in the hopes that it may assist the fitness professional better convey nutrition information to their clients. On the following page is an example of a typical food label. For this example, a box of cereal was chosen but in general, all food labels will have the same basic look. Let's now examine the various parts of the typical food label.

Serving Size

All food labels begin with the words "Nutrition Facts" at the top. Directly below this will be the *serving size* that is recommended and *servings per container that the package contains*. By law, food labels must tell us what the serving size is in both metric units as well as a more *understandable* unit of measure. In the example depicted here, we see that a serving size is 1¼ of a cup and this is equal to 30 grams. Government regulations also require that the serving size be standardized. In other words, you won't see two brands of bread or two kinds of soda with different serving sizes. Serving size is predetermined to help the consumer make easy comparisons between different brands of the same type of food. Food labels must also specify the *number of servings* that the package of food contains. In the example used here, the label indicates that the package contains about 13 servings. This means that if you measured all of the 1¼ cup serving sizes contained in this example, there would be about 13 servings

Some nutrition labels contain a little trick that involves serving sizes. Nutrition labels are based on one serving only— but there may be two or more servings per container! For example, a serving size of soda is typically eight ounces, and the calories, etc. on the nutrition label are based on only eight ounces. Yet a 20 ounce bottle of soda contains 2 ½ servings per container. Thus, the calories, etc. on the label must be multiplied by 2.5 to arrive at the *real* amounts it contains!

NUTRITION FACTS

Serving Size 1 ¼ cup (30g)
Servings per container about 13

Amount per serving	Cereal	Cereal with ½ cup of skim milk
Calories	200	240
Calories from fat	10	10
		% Daily Value**
Total Fat 1.0g*	2%	2%
Saturated Fat 0g	0%	0%
Trans Fat 0g		
Polyunsaturated Fat 0.5		
Monounsaturated Fat 0g		
Cholesterol 0mg	0%	0%
Sodium 0mg	0%	3%
Potassium 85mg	2%	8%
Total carbohydrate 47g	16%	18%
Dietary Fiber 5g	20%	20%
Soluble Fiber less than 1 g		
Insoluble Fiber 5g		
Sugars 11g		
Protein 5g		
Vitamin A	25%	30%
Vitamin C	25%	25%
Calcium	0%	4%
Iron	2%	15%
Folate	25%	25%

*Amount in cereal
** Percent Daily Values are based on a 2,000 calorie diet.
   Your daily values may be higher or lower depending on your calorie needs.

	Calories:	2,000	2,500
Total fat	less than	65g	80g
Sat fat	less than	20g	25g
Cholesterol	less than	300mg	300mg
Sodium	less than	2,300mg	2,300mg
Potassium		3,500mg	3,500mg
Total Carbohydrate		300g	375g
Dietary Fiber		25g	30g

Calories per gram:
Fat 9   *   Carbohydrate 4   *   Protein 4

118

The serving size used in this example also tells us that we would have to eat 30 grams of this product (or 1¼ cup if you prefer) to get the amounts of calories, fat, carbohydrate, cholesterol, sodium, fiber, sugar and protein listed on the label. Thus, all of the nutrient levels on the label are also based on a single serving size.

Calories

Next, is the calorie content of the food. In this example, we see that the food contains 200 calories by itself—and 240 calories if we consume it with ½ cup of skim milk. Directly below calories is the amount of *calories from fat.* Here we see that 10 calories are derived from fat if the cereal is eaten dry and 10 calories if consumed with ½ cup of skim milk. Skim milk has negligible amounts of fat so hence the reason this value doesn't change.

Total Fat

The Total Fat section of the food label indicates the total amount of fat that is contained in a serving size. In this example, the total fat is 1 gram (1 gram of fat has 9 calories which is rounded to 10 calories in the previous section, "calories from fat"). We also see that this one gram of total fat represents 2 percent of our *daily value* for fat (more on *daily value* later). Below Total Fat are the gram amounts of fat coming from *Saturated, Polyunsaturated* and *Monounsaturated* fat. Trans fat is also now listed on food labels because of evidence that they are linked to heart disease.

Cholesterol

Cholesterol must also be listed on all food labels. In the present example, we see that the food contains zero milligrams of cholesterol per serving.

Sodium & Potassium

Just under the reference for cholesterol are listings for sodium and potassium, two other ingredients that must be listed on all food labels. In the example used here, we see that this particular food contains zero milligrams of sodium and 85 milligrams of potassium.

Total Carbohydrate

Food labels must also indicate the total amount of carbohydrate that a serving of the food contains. In the current example, a serving contains 47 grams of carbohydrate. Total carbohydrate is an all inclusive category and includes sugars which are also listed separately to help people differentiate how much of the total carbs is contributed specifically by sugar.

Dietary Fiber

Because high fiber diets are linked to reduced risk of various diseases, food labels also list this nutrient as well. In the present example we see that a serving size contains 5 grams of fiber. Below dietary fiber are the gram amounts for both soluble (less than 1 gram) and insoluble fiber (5 grams). Both soluble and insoluble fiber appear to have different effects in the body. Soluble fiber has been shown to help lower cholesterol levels while insoluble fiber gives food bulk and may help people feel fuller longer.

Sugar

Food labels must also list the gram amounts per serving size for sugar which in this example is 11 grams. Sugar is a simple carbohydrate and is usually listed separate from Total Carbohydrates described previously. This is because all carbohydrates are not created equal. Sugars, like table sugar, tend to raise blood glucose levels fast and generally do not contain many nutrients. Complex carbohydrates are more nutrient-dense and raise blood glucose levels slower and as such are considered healthier than simple sugars. It's possible to have a lot of carbohydrates yet have little or even zero sugars in a food. Notice also that there is no *daily value* listed for sugars. This is because sugar does not have any specific recommendations for intake. This is contrasted by Total Carbohydrates which does have a daily value.

Protein

Keeping track of how much protein somebody eats is pretty easy because all food labels list this amount. In the present example, the food label indicates 5 grams of protein per serving. There is no RDA for protein.

Vitamins and Minerals

By law, food labels must list the percent daily values for vitamin A, vitamin C, calcium, and iron. Other vitamins and minerals may also be listed on the food label although this is not mandatory.

What are Daily Values?

Most who read food labels have probably noticed a lot of percentages for the different nutrients—these are the daily values (DVs). Daily values represent suggested nutrient intake levels that are appropriate for most individuals, regardless of age or gender. For example, on the food label used here, we see that each serving of product contains 47 grams of carbohydrate and that this represents 16% of our daily value for this nutrient. The daily values—which are based on the RDA's—were adopted because RDAs can fluctuate according to age and gender as well as other conditions. Thus, daily values are meant to help make reading food labels easier. The daily values listed for the nutrients on food labels are based a 2000 calorie per day diet. Close to the bottom of food labels you will also see the daily values of several nutrients listed for someone consuming a 2500 calorie per day diet. Both 2000 and 2500 calorie diets were chosen so as to make the food label more applicable to the diets of most Americans. In other words, the reasoning was that most Americans consume somewhere between 2000 and 2500 calories a day. Below are the daily values of some of the more important nutrients. These values are also listed at the bottom of most food labels as well.

Daily Values (Based on a 2000 calorie diet)	
Nutrient	Daily Value
Total Fat	65 grams
Saturated Fat	20 grams
Cholesterol	300 milligrams
Total Carbohydrate	300 grams
Dietary Fiber	25 grams
Sodium	2300 milligrams
Potassium	3500 milligrams
Protein	50 grams

Calories per Gram

At the very bottom of most food labels are the calories that are contained in a gram of fat, carbohydrate and protein (9, 4 and 4 calories respectively). These numbers can be used to calculate the actual number of calories from fat, carbohydrate and protein in a serving size of the food in question. For example, on the food label used here, we see that the total carbohydrate in one serving is 47 grams. Since each gram of carbohydrate contains 4 calories, this means that 47 X 4 = 188 calories from carbohydrate are in one serving. If we wanted to know what percent of the food was carbohydrate, we would divide the calories from carbohydrates (188) by the total calories in a serving (200). This would equal 188/200 = 94% carbohydrate. Thus, the food in this example, is about 94% carbohydrate per serving. These same calculations can be done for fat and protein.

Food Label Buzz Words

In the past, food labels could say almost anything they wanted. This is no longer so and the regulations that govern what can and cannot be claimed on food labels are very specific. What follows is a summary of the major allowable food label claims and what they mean.

- **Fat Free.** In order for a product to post the label that its "fat free", it must either have zero fat—or contain an insignificant amount of fat (usually defined as less than ½ gram per serving).

- **Low Fat.** Foods that make the claim that they are "low fat" can only do so if they contain less than 3 grams of fat per serving size.

- **Low in Saturated Fat.** A food that is low in saturated fat must contain less than 1 gram of saturated fat per serving.

- **Cholesterol Free.** To be called cholesterol free, the food in question must contain less than 2 milligrams of cholesterol per serving size.

- **Calorie Free.** By law, only foods that contain less than 5 calories per serving can make the calorie free claim. So, technically, even calorie free foods have some calories.

- **Sodium Free.** Foods listed as sodium free can only do so if they contain less than 2 milligrams of sodium per serving.

- **Light (or Lite).** For a food package to make the claim that it is *light*, it must contain either a *third less calories* or *one half less fat* than that contained in the original recipe of the product. Beware. It's possible for a food to make this claim yet still contain high amounts of fat. For example, suppose the original recipe had 99g of fat and the light version has 1/3rd less. That means that the light version has 66 grams of fat. That's the entire daily value for fat! Rule of thumb: do the math yourself when you see this claim.

- **Healthy.** For a product to use the word "Healthy", it must provide at least 10% of the daily value per serving of either or all of the following: vitamin A, vitamin C, calcium, iron, fiber or protein. In addition, each serving must contain no more than 60 mg of cholesterol or no more than 480 mg sodium.

- **Good Source.** A food can be labeled a "good source" of various nutrients if the food contains between 10-19% more than the daily value of the nutrient in question. In addition, there must be scientific evidence showing that the nutrient in question has health benefits. For example, evidence suggests that folate can lower birth defects. Thus, foods high in folate can be said to be a *good source* of this vitamin. If there is no proof of health benefits associated with elevated levels of a nutrient, then the *good source* claim cannot be made. Other terms for good source that also show up on food labels include "high" "rich in" and "excellent source".

- **Reduced.** For a food label to make the reduced claim, it must contain at least 25% less calories, fat, saturated fat, cholesterol, sodium or sugar than the original recipe for the product. So if the original recipe had 100 grams of total fat, then the *reduced* claim could be made if the new version of the product had 75 grams of fat per serving.

- ***Organic.*** According the USDA, the term "organic" means that a food was grown without synthetic fertilizers, or the use of biotechnology or radiation. Most pesticides are also banned from being used with organic foods. In 2002 the US department of Agriculture launched its official federal guidelines by which foods could call themselves "organic". According to these guidelines three terms may now be displayed on foods: The terms and their definitions are below:

  - **"100% Organic"** means that all of a products ingredients are organic.

  - **"Organic"** is different than 100% organic and means that at least 95% of a products ingredients are organic.

  - **"Made with Organic Ingredients"** means that the product has at least 70% organically derived ingredients

- ***Natural.*** Despite showing up frequently on food labels, the word "natural" has no legal definition. As such, it carries much less weight than *organic, healthy* or other words mentioned in this section. In theory, a food that only bears the "natural" label could be high in saturated fat, trans fat or other compounds that most people associate with being unhealthy.

Chapter 15

Questions & Answers

Fitness professionals are always being asked questions about health, wellness, exercise and even to help make sense of health reports appearing in magazines, TV and radio. This chapter is about not only those questions but also questions that fitness professionals themselves may be asking but having trouble finding straight answers.

Q. Are beans a *good* source of protein?
A. Yes and no. Beans provide protein but do not provide full spectrum of essential amino acids. Thus, while they are a good source of protein, they are not "high quality" protein like chicken, fish, etc. This is why vegetarians often combine beans and rice together with meals.

Q. What is gluten?
A. Gluten is a protein found in products containing wheat, rye or barley. As such it shows up frequently in the foods we eat. People with the digestive disorder, celiac disease, have a problem digesting gluten. In these people (which could be 1 in every 133 Americans according to some reports) gluten provokes the immune system which then inflames and damages the small intestine, causing people distress. Some research links celiac disease with the development of type I diabetes, rheumatoid arthritis and other disorders. After celiac disease is diagnosed by a physician, the person should avoid foods that contain gluten.

Q. How do people lose weight on low carb diets?
A. When a person starts a low carbohydrate diet, they will likely lose a large amount of weight within the first couple of weeks. The main reason for this has to do with glycogen, which is the body's storage form of sugar. When we significantly reduce the amount of carbohydrates we eat, our body begins to degrade its glycogen reserves in order to keep our blood sugar from falling too much (we can die if blood sugar gets to low!). As glycogen is utilized, a lot of water is released in the process. In fact, for every gram of glycogen that is used, roughly three grams of water are freed up! The body has to do something with all that water so it sends people to the bathroom to get rid of it. Thus, for the first few weeks, most of the weight that is lost on a low carb diet is in the form of water. Another reason stems from the limited variety of foods eaten on such diets. Research shows that people eat more when they have a variety of foods to chose from and eat less when there are fewer chooses. Cutting carbs reduces the choices on these diets. That cuts out additional calories and probably leads to further weight loss.

Q. What is a normal level for cholesterol?

A. Currently a total cholesterol level of less than 200 mg/dl is considered normal / healthy for adults. In addition people should strive for their LDL to be less than 100 mg/dl. Triglycerides should be less than 150 mg/dl. With respect to HDL, greater than 40 mg/dl is advisable. In fact an HDL of 60 mg/dl or more is often called a "negative risk factor" for heart disease (that is, it reduces heart disease risk). While weight loss often can sometimes improve cholesterol levels, exercise, especially aerobic exercise, helps raise HDL levels.

Q. How is total cholesterol calculated? Is it just the HDL + LDL?

A. Total cholesterol is found by this equation: Total cholesterol = HDL+ LDL + (triglycerides ÷5). For example, If your HDL is 50, your LDL is 80 and your triglycerides are 60, your total cholesterol is found this way:

        Step 1. HDL +LDL = 50 + 80 = 130.

        Step 2. Divide the triglycerides by 5: 60 ÷5 = 12.

        Step 3. Total cholesterol = 130 + 12 = **142**

Q. What is the difference between an RD and a nutritionist?

A. A registered dietitian (RD) is someone who has at least a BS degree in nutrition and has passed the American Dietetics Association certification test. Most also do an internship under the tutelage of another qualified dietitian. A *nutritionist* is a more general term that may or may not refer to an RD. Some dietitians do refer to themselves as nutritionists. But, depending on the state in which one resides, the term nutritionist might be used by almost anyone—including those with no formal nutrition education or certification.

Q. Can personal trainers give nutrition advice?

A. Laws may differ from state to state. Fitness professionals are encouraged to visit their local county government or consult their legal professional for the laws in their area. For those who work at health clubs, additional rules may also apply. Some health clubs may have specific staff associates whom they refer members to for nutrition-related information. Regardless of issues of legality and internal health club policies, fitness professionals should strive network with nutrition professionals like registered dietitians (RDs). Dietitians undoubtedly have clients that are trying to lose weight and need to exercise and personal trainers usually have a number of clients they could refer to a dietician for help with nutrition. As a rule, dietitians know nutrition, not proper exercise technique. This is a void that an alliance with a personal trainer could fill very well. Together both fitness professional and dietitian might be more effective at helping people than either one could be by themselves. For a list of dietitians in your area, fitness professionals can look in the telephone book or visit the American Dietetic Association website, www. eatright.org

Q. Can someone be a vegetarian and still eat meat?

A. Yes. Some vegetarians do in fact eat meat occasionally. These individuals fall into a category sometimes called "flexitarians" which essentially means they are *flexible* in their food choices and sometimes eat meat because they recognize that there is no one perfect food. Eating meat is also an easy way to make sure they are getting complete proteins in their diet. As a rule, flexitarians do not make meat the main portion of their meals but rather the meat they consume compliments the other foods that they eat during the day.

Q. Can people lose fat in just certain areas?
A. Unfortunately, with the exception of liposuction, it is not possible to lose fat from only specific areas of the body. This fallacy is referred to as "spot reduction" and ironically is the premise behind many weight loss gizmos advertised on TV. If spot reduction worked, one would expect to see less fat on the dominant arms of tennis players and baseball pitchers, who typically exercise one limb more than the other. But this isn't what is observed. The pattern that is seen is that when we exercise, we lose fat all over the body at the same time. So you will lose fat from under your arms, your thighs, tummy, around your internal organs and even from your little pinky finger! Overall, this is far more of a healthier way to lose excess body fat.

Q. What does partially hydrogenated mean?
A. To hydrogenate a fat means to add hydrogen atoms to it. This changes the chemical properties of the fat. Saturated fats are literally *saturated* with hydrogen atoms. Partially hydrogenated, while less saturated with hydrogen is nevertheless also a saturated fat. Another phrase that is also used on food labels is "tropical oils". Tropical oils, like palm oil, palm kernel oil and coconut oil are also saturated fats. Saturated fats are implicated in the development of heart disease and as such are things to avoid as much as possible. Specifically, saturated fats have been shown to raise LDL (bad cholesterol). Considering how harmful they are, some might wonder why they are used in the first place. Well, saturated fats do help increase the shelf life of a food which in turn keeps the price down. Think how expensive cookies and cakes might be if they spoiled after a few days! So, from an economical viewpoint saturated fats make sense but from a health viewpoint they are things to avoid. While partially hydrogenated fats contain less hydrogen atoms, they are likely to possess more trans fats which were discussed earlier in this book.

Q. What are sugar alcohols?
A. While technically neither a sugar or an alcohol, sugar alcohols are molecules that *look* like both sugars and alcohols. Because they tend to contain fewer calories than regular sugar (1.5 to 3 calories per gram as opposed to 4 calories per gram for sugar), sugar alcohols are often used in place of sugar in low calorie and low carb foods and as well as in some nutritional supplements. Common sugar alcohols include mannitol, sorbitol, and xylitol. Another difference between traditional carbohydrates and sugar alcohols is that sugar alcohols don't raise insulin levels very much, if at all. Thus, sugar alcohols may also be found in diabetic foods as well. Sugar alcohols do not contain any alcohol like the kind found in alcoholic beverages so they will not make people drunk.

Q. What is the difference between the Daily Values (DV) and Dietary Reference intakes (DRI)?

A. The daily values (DV) that are listed on food labels in the US are not age or gender dependant unlike the DRIs which are. The DRIs are essentially a revamping of the RDAs and are for the most part used by nutrition and health professionals. Because the DRIs contain 4 values (i.e. the RDA, EAR, AI and UL, which were defined in a previous chapter), they may cause confusion among those not in the health, wellness or nutrition field. To clarify this and make things easier for the general public, the FDA mandated that food labels list an easier to understand reference for consumers - the Daily Values.

Q. What does the "L" on amino acid supplement labels mean?

A. The letter L that is on the labels of amino acid supplements is a chemistry term that essentially means the molecules are "left handed". Molecules, like people, can be either right-handed or left-handed. It turns out that all the essential and non-essential amino acids in the human body are left handed. Hence the amino acid names like
L arginine, L glutamine, etc.

Q. What are "healthy" trans fats?

A. Fitness professionals often find themselves on the front lines of fielding a multitude of questions as they help people make sense of health and wellness-related information. The case for trans fats is a classic example of this. When used in excess, research finds that trans fats tend to increase the risk of heart disease. In recent years though there has been speculation if some trans fats might promote health and fight disease. One example of this issue is conjugated linoleic acid (CLA), where emerging research hints may have anti-cancer properties.[73] Naturally occurring trans fats might also be processed differently artificial trans fats. At this point, nobody is suggesting that any type of trans fat prevents cancer in humans and the notion of "healthy" trans fats is a controversial topic. This highlights though the need for fitness professionals to stay on top of health-related information.

Q. Do we have to exercise for 20 minutes before burning fat?

A. The statement that we must exercise for 20 to 30 minutes before we begin to use our fat reserves is popular among some fitness experts. In reality however, we are always burning fat, it's just a matter of how much we are talking about. At rest, roughly 60% of the energy being burned is coming from fat, while about 40% stems from carbohydrate burning. When exercise starts, we begin to burn more carbs and less fat. However, as we continue to exercise, a gradual shift occurs where we begin using less carbs and more fat. So, do we have to exercise for at lest 20 minutes before we start the fat burning process? Technically no, but after 20 minutes of exercise we are using a lot more fat than we are after only one minute of exercise. Also, the longer one exercises, the more calories are burned.

Q. Can we drink too much water?

A. Yes. A condition exists where individuals consume so much water during exercise that they may suffer life-threatening symptoms. This condition is called *hyponatremia* (pronounced, hypo-nay-tree-me-ah). Hyponatremia results when water is consumed in such excess that it dilutes the concentration of the body's sodium and other electrolytes. Remember that sodium (along with potassium) plays a major role in facilitating both muscle contraction and the transmission of nerve impulses. Sodium is also responsible for keeping the body's fluid levels at their proper concentrations. As fluid levels increase (by drinking water), the concentration of sodium and other electrolytes actually decreases as it is dispersed through a greater volume of fluid. This, coupled with sodium losses through sweat, can lead to life-threatening consequences. Some evidence suggests that the body can only eliminate about one quart of water per hour. Thus, consuming two or more quarts per hour during exercise could, in theory, lead to hyponatremia.

While typically observed in those who compete in long-endurance events like marathons and triathlons, hyponatremia may also occur in other events as well such as football or the pre-season training for such sports—where the individual may not be accustomed to the rigors of exercise and may be more likely to consume large volumes of water. Treatment of hyponatremia requires immediate medical attention and involves intravenous sodium replacement. Symptoms of hyponatremia including swollen feet and hands, nausea, vomiting, and confusion/disorientation to name a few. One possible sign that hyponatremia may occur is weight gain immediately following exercise. Normally one would expect an individual to lose weight after exercise due to fluid losses from sweat. Weight gain immediately after exercise may indicate that the person is consuming too much water. While this observation is not foolproof, noticing weight gain after exercise may allow the fitness professional an opportunity to discuss hyponatremia with their clients. The goal here is not to frighten individuals to not drink any water, but rather to make them aware of a situation which may occur during excessive fluid consumption.

Q. Are natural vitamins better than synthetic vitamins?
A. Technically the body does not know the difference between synthetic vitamins made in the laboratory and natural vitamins, made in nature. This is because the chemical structures of synthetic and natural vitamins are identical.

The case for vitamin E is one classic example often used in an attempt to prove the superiority of natural over synthetic vitamins. It turns out that the body does in fact utilize natural vitamin E better than synthetic vitamin E—and for a very good reason. Some people in the world are left-handed and others are right-handed. The same is also true for molecules as well! Technically, we refer to left-handed molecules as *levorotory* (or L for short). Right-handed molecules are given the name *dextrorotatory* (or d for short). The human body prefers right-handed (d) vitamin E over left-hand (L) vitamin E. So in theory, natural vitamin E would be composed of all right-handed molecules (in other words, only the d version). Synthetic vitamin E is actually composed of a mixture of both right and left-handed molecules (referred to as "dl alpha tocopherol" on many multivitamin labels). But we can only use the right handed (d) version. So, theoretically, only 50% of synthetic vitamin E can be utilized by the body. It should be noted however, right-handed vitamin E made in the laboratory, is absorbed no differently than right-handed vitamin E made in nature's *laboratory*.

Q. Why are multivitamins usually low in calcium?

A. Many multivitamins provide a percentage of the RDA for calcium. The reason for this is because calcium is a pretty big molecule. Stuffing the entire RDA into a single multivitamin in addition to all the other nutrients would make the vitamin even bigger than it already is. The bulkiness of the calcium molecule is also the reason why calcium supplements tend to be so big.

Q. When using creatine supplements is the "loading" phase needed?

A. When creatine first came to public attention, everybody was advocating that people begin with what was called a "loading phase" whereby 20-25 grams a day of creatine would be used for the first week of supplementation. This was then to be followed by a "maintenance phase" that consisted of only 2-5 grams a day. But is the loading phase needed to reap the benefits of creatine? Apparently it isn't. In a study published in the *Journal of Applied Physiology*, researchers found that 28 days of using 3 grams of creatine per day enhanced muscle creatine reserves as well as did 20 grams per day for a week.[129] The take home message seems clear; if you are not in a hurry, loading creatine is not needed. For more on creatine, read my book *Nutritional Supplements*, available at my website www.Joe-Cannon.com

Q. When is the best time to take vitamins?

A. While there is no "best" or perfect time but as a rule it's probably best to take multivitamins with food. The reason for this is that when you eat, you produce more stomach acid which helps with absorption. In addition, because a meal probably contains some fat, this will also facilitate the absorption of the fat soluble vitamins (A, E, D & K) as well.

Q. What's better: protein before or after exercise?

A. Both strategies have merit. Eating some protein (and carbs) 2-3 hrs before a workout can help supply the body with nutrients needed during training. That being said this practice may cause cramping or GI problems for some, especially those who eat a big meal just prior to exercise. Research also suggests that consuming protein (and carbs) immediately (i.e. within 1 hour) after exercise appears to be superior at building muscle to eating several hours after exercise. [141] The enzyme glycogen synthase (which makes glycogen) is most active for about an hour after exercise. Since carbs help with the assimilation of amino acids via the action of insulin, this may be another reason to eat protein (and carbs) after exercise. Besides elite athletes, this issue may be especially important to older adults who may grapple with sarcopenia need to pay the most attention to this issue.

Glossary

Adipose Tissue. Adipose is another name for fat tissue. Triglycerides are stored in adipose tissue.

Aerobic Exercise. Exercise that uses oxygen as a means to generate energy (ATP). Also any exercise that you can do for a prolonged period of time without stopping. Usually during aerobic exercise, fat is used as a fuel source. Examples include, walking, swimming, bike riding and jogging.

AI. A nutrition term which stands for *adequate intake*. Adequate intakes for nutrients are used by nutrition professionals when there is not enough evidence available for determination of an RDA. See also RDA and UL

Amenorrhea. The cessation of menstrual cycles. May occur in anorexia nervosa. See also oligomenorrhea.

Amino Acid. The building blocks of proteins. There are twenty amino acids that the body uses to make proteins. Amino acids can be divided into essential (which we must obtain from food) and non-essential (which our bodies can make on their own) amino acids. See also proteins.

Anabolism. Refers to the buildup or synthesis of substances in the body. See also catabolism.

Anaerobic Exercise. Exercise that does not require oxygen to help with the generation of energy (ATP). Examples are weight lifting, powerlifting and sprinting.

Antioxidant. Any substance that reduces the production of free radicals. Vitamins E and C are two classic examples of antioxidants. See also free radical.

ATP. Adenosine Triphosphate. ATP is the body's ultimate energy molecule. ATP is an immediate source of energy for muscle contraction. The energy (calories) in the food is rearranged into a usable form of energy – ATP.

Bioelectric Impedance Analysis. A method of body composition determination that uses a small electric current that passes through the body. Sometimes abbreviated as BIA. See also hydrostatic weighing.

BMR. Basal Metabolic Rate. The lowest metabolism possible. See also RMR.

Body Composition. The amount of fat and fat-free mass that a body contains.

Body Mass Index. A relatively quick way to assess body composition. Abbreviated as BMI. BMI is equal to a person's weight in kilograms divided by height in meters squared (BMI = weight (kg) / height (m^2)). As BMI increases, so too does risk for obesity-related disease.

Calorie. A calorie is a unit of heat energy. Specifically, the amount of heat needed to raise 1 kilogram of water (1 liter) 1 degree Celsius. Calories are the key to weight loss and weight gain. Consuming more calories than are expended through exercise and daily activities results in weight gain. Consuming fewer calories than are expended through exercise and daily activities results in weight loss. Calories are derived from three macronutrients— proteins, carbohydrates and fats. Other synonymous names for calorie include kilogram calorie, Kcal and kilocalorie.

Carbohydrate. Carbohydrates are sugars. Carbohydrates are the primary energy source used during exercise. Every gram of carbohydrate has 4 calories. Food sources of carbohydrates include breads, cereals, pasta, rice, etc.

Cardiovascular Exercise. Any exercise that one can do for a prolonged period of time without stopping. Examples include walking, hiking, jogging, swimming, and bike riding. It is also called aerobic exercise.

Catabolism. Refers to the breaking down of a substance in the body. See also anabolism.

Cholesterol. A substance made in the liver that is indispensable for life. Too much though can build up in the body and eventually contribute to diseases such as high blood pressure, strokes and heart attacks. *See also HDL and LDL cholesterol.*

Complete Protein. Also called high quality protein. A complete protein source contains all of the essential amino acids in the proper amounts for humans. Meats, poultry and fish are good sources of complete proteins.

Creatine Phosphate. Creatine is an energy source that the body uses to regenerate ATP during periods of intense physical activity like sprinting or heavy weight lifting. Creatine is found in meat and fish products and is also naturally produced in the body.

Diabetes. A disease in which the body either does not make insulin or cannot make use of the insulin that is present. Diabetes is divided into Type I, where the person does not make insulin (so, insulin must be injected daily) and Type II, where the individual can not make use of the insulin that is made. Overweight individuals are at risk for both types of diabetes.

Dietary Supplement. Defined as any substance *for use by man to supplement the diet by increasing the total dietary intake.* Includes but is not limited to vitamins, minerals, herbs, some hormones, amino acids and enzymes, to name a few.

DNA. Stands for "de-oxy-ribo-nucleic acid". Our genetic material. DNA is a "blueprint" or software program of how to make another you. The chromosomes are made of DNA.

DRI. Dietary reference intake. A nutrition term that was created when the RDA was revamped.

Enzyme. A biological catalyst. Enzymes are biological *machines* that speed up chemical reactions and help them occur faster than they normally would. Practically every chemical reaction in the body requires an enzyme. Enzymes are manufactured in the body and can be used over again many times before wearing out. When an enzyme finally wears out, an identical enzyme is made.

Ephedra. Ephedra is the herb which contains the drug ephedrine, which mimics the effect of adrenaline in the body. Also called Ma-Huang. Side effects of ephedra can include increased heart rate and blood pressure and possibly death.

Ergogenic Aid. Ergogenic aids refer to any substance or product that is touted to enhance exercise ability. Examples of ergogenic aids include creatine, caffeine, androstendione and even some clothing products to name a few.

Essential. In reference to nutrition, essential refers to a substance which must be consumed in the diet. For example, essential amino acids are essential because we cannot make them and thus must obtain them from food or supplements.

Fat. Fat is the body's long-term energy storage molecule. Every gram of fat has 9 calories (in contrast, protein and carbohydrate only have about 4 calories per gram). One pound of fat contains 3500 calories.

Fiber. The name given to indigestible carbohydrates derived from plants. Fiber can be subdivided into soluble fiber and insoluble fiber.

Free Radical. A molecule or atom which can disrupt normal cellular functioning. Free radicals are produced by normal cellular activities and are normally kept in check by antioxidant defense systems as well as foods which contain antioxidants. In excess, however, it is theorized that free radicals may contribute to a wide variety of diseases and syndromes such as cancer. It is not possible to completely rid the body of free radicals. *See also antioxidant.*

Gene. A region of DNA which contains genetic instructions for specific traits such as eye color, muscle fiber type or bone density. *See also DNA.*

Glucose. Blood sugar. Normal blood sugar is < 100 mg/dl. *See also glycogen and glycolysis.*

Glycogen. Another form of carbohydrate. Glycogen is made up of sugar (specifically, glucose). The body stores a certain amount of sugar for use during exercise and during periods of non-eating. This sugar is called glycogen. It is from this term that we get the word glycolysis. *See also glycolysis.*

Glycolysis. The chemical pathway responsible for the breakdown of sugar (glucose) for energy (ATP) that does not require oxygen. Glycolysis is an anaerobic energy generating pathway. Generally, as exercise intensity increases, so too does glycolysis. A byproduct of glycolysis is lactic acid, which causes a *burning* sensation inside the muscles as well as muscle fatigue. *See also ATP, glycogen and glucose.*

Gram. Unit of weight in the metric system. There are about 28 grams in one ounce. *See also protein, fat and carbohydrate.*

HDL. The so-called "good" cholesterol. HDL (high density lipoprotein) is a molecule that transports cholesterol. HDL transports cholesterol from the blood, back to the liver where it is broken down. It is advantageous to have a high level of HDL in your blood in light of evidence that HDL can help reduce the risk of heart disease. On blood tests, HDL should be 40 mg/dl or better. *See also LDL and cholesterol.*

Hormone. A chemical messenger. The body contains many hormones such as testosterone, estrogen, and insulin. Hormones regulate many biological processes.

Hydrogenation. The process of making a saturated fat from an unsaturated fat. During the hydrogenation process, a fat is *saturated* with hydrogen atoms. High intakes of saturated fats are linked to heart disease. *See also saturated and unsaturated fat.*

Hypercholesterolemia. Another name for high cholesterol levels. *See also cholesterol, HDL and LDL.*

Hypertension. High blood pressure. Hypertension is blood pressure that is chronically above 140/90 mm Hg. The letters "mm Hg" stand for millimeters of mercury". Hypertension is sometimes abbreviated as HTN. Hypertension places one at greater risk of heart disease.

Ketone. A molecule formed during severe calorie or carbohydrate restriction. Ketones can act as an alternative energy source for many of the body's cells. Excessive ketone formation (ketosis) is dangerous in that they alter the chemistry of the body (i.e. decreases pH, which increases acidity of the body). This, in turn, negatively affects normal body functions. *See also pH.*

Kilogram. A metric system unit of measurement. One kilogram = 1,000 grams. One kilogram (or 1 kg) is equal to about 2.2 pounds.

Krebs Cycle. The name given to the chemical reaction that involves the aerobic breakdown of fat. The Krebs cycle occurs in the mitochondria. Other names for the Krebs cycle include the TCA cycle (tricarboxylic acid cycle) and the citric acid cycle. *See also mitochondria, fat, carbohydrate and glycolysis.*

Lactic Acid. A metabolic byproduct of glycolysis made during the anaerobic breaking down sugar (glucose) for energy (ATP). Elevations in lactic acid alter the pH of cells and are cause the burning sensation in muscles during intense exercise.

LDL. The so-called "bad" cholesterol. LDL (low density lipoprotein) is a molecule that transports cholesterol. LDL transports cholesterol from where it is made out to the cells of the body where it can be used. High levels of LDL in the blood are deemed a contributor of heart disease.

Lean Body Mass. Traditionally, lean body mass (LBM) has been used to refer to muscle mass. Lean body mass is anything in the body other than fat mass. Thus, LBM also includes bone and water.

Lipid. Another name for fat.

Macronutrient. Nutrients that make up the greatest amount of our diet. Proteins, fats and carbohydrates are the macronutrients. *See also protein, fat and carbohydrate.*

MET. Stands for metabolic equivalents. One MET is equal to 3.5 milliliters of oxygen per kilogram of body weight per minute. METs are another way to measure exercise intensity. An exercise intensity of 3 METs is three times more difficult as an intensity of 1 MET. *See also oxygen consumption and VO_2.*

Metabolism. The total of all the building-up chemical reactions (anabolic reactions) and breaking-down chemical reactions (catabolic reactions) in the body. Metabolism can also be thought of as the speed at which we burn calories. Faster metabolisms burn calories faster than slower metabolisms.

Mitochondria. A region of the cell where fat is broken down to generate energy (ATP). Aerobic exercise can stimulate production of more mitochondria. *See also fat and Krebs cycle.*

Non-Essential. With regard to nutrition, a substance that does not need to be obtained from food or supplements. In other words, the body can produce the substance on its own. Non-essential amino acids are examples of non-essential nutrients. *See also amino acid.*

Oligomenorrhea. Irregular menstrual cycles. May be observed in bulimia nervosa. *See also amenorrhea.*

Osteoporosis. A disease where bones become brittle and break easily. Osteoporosis can affect not only women but men also. Bone loss begins around the age of 35.

Peer-Reviewed. A scientific study is peer-reviewed when it is first reviewed by other competent scientists (peers) prior to publication. This decreases errors in the study which might have occurred and allows for a better study better. Articles printed in popular magazines and newspapers are generally not peer-reviewed.

pH. Refers to an acidity scale that is commonly used in science. The scale runs from zero-14. A pH of seven is considered neutral. The lower the number on the pH scale, the more acid a substance is. Overall, the pH of the human body is about 7.35.

Phosphagen. A high-energy containing molecule. ATP and phosphocreatine are examples of the phosphagens.

Phytonutrients. Nutrients derived from fruits and vegetables. Also called phytochemicals.

Protein. One of the macronutrients. Protein contains 4 calories/gram. Proteins are made of smaller units called amino acids. *See also amino acid.*

RDA. Recommended Dietary Allowance. The RDA's represent nutrient intakes in amounts needed to ward off diseases associated with nutrient deficiencies.

Registered Dietitian. A registered dietitian (RD) is a nutrition professional who has at the very least a bachelor's degree in nutrition and who has passed the American Dietetic Association (ADA) examination.

RMR. Resting Metabolic Rate. The minimum amount of calories needed to sustain the vital functions of the body. RMR is proportional to body size. Thus, taller, heavier people will have a higher RMR than do shorter, lighter people. Resting metabolic rate tends to decrease by 2-5% per decade after age 40. *See also BMR.*

Saturated Fat. A saturated fat is saturated with hydrogen atoms. Saturated fats are more unhealthy than unsaturated fats. Saturated fats tend to be solid at room temperature.

Sedentary. A term that refers to minimal physical activity.

Trans Fatty Acid. Refers to the molecular arrangement of the atoms which make up a fat. Trans fatty acids are usually made when saturated fats are made. Some research shows that some trans fatty acids may be detrimental to health by fostering heart disease. *See also saturated fat, unsaturated fat, HDL, LDL and cholesterol.*

Triglyceride. Another name for fat. Triglycerides are stored in fat cells and are released into the blood when needed such as during aerobic exercise. *See also adipose tissue.*

UL. A nutrition term which stands for *tolerable upper intake level.* It refers to the highest level of a nutrient that can be safely consumed. Intakes above the UL increase the potential that negative side effects might occur. *See also AI, DRI and RDA.*

Unsaturated Fat. Unsaturated fats tend to be liquid at room temperature and are more heart-healthy. Unsaturated fats are not as saturated with hydrogen atoms compared to saturated fats. Monounsaturated fats and polyunsaturated fats refer to the degree of saturation. *See also saturated fat.*

Vitamin. An organic substance needed in small amounts by the body to help sustain life processes. Vitamins can be divided into water-soluble vitamins (B complex and vitamin C) and fat-soluble vitamins (A, D, E & K). *See also mineral.*

VO$_2$. Abbreviation for volume of oxygen. VO$_2$ used as a measure of exercise intensity and aerobic fitness. *See also oxygen consumption and METs.*

References

1. ACSM Position Stand (2001). Appropriate intervention strategies for weight loss and prevention of weight regain in adults Medicine and Science in Sports and Exercise, 33, 12, 2145-2156.

2. ACSM (2000). ACSM's Guidelines for Exercise Testing and Prescription, 6th edition. Lippincott, Williams and Wilkins.

3. ACSM Position Stand (1997). Female Athletic Triad. Medicine and Science in Sports and Exercise, 29, 5, pp. i-ix.

4. Adebowale, A. O. et al. (2000). Analysis of glucosamine and chondroitin sulfate content in marketed products and the caco-2 permeability of chondroitin sulfate raw materials. Journal of the American Nutraceutical Association,3, 1, 37-44.

5. Alexander, J. L. (2002). The role of resistance exercise in weight loss. Strength & Conditioning Journal, 24, 11, 65-69.

6. Arner, P. et al. (1990). Expression of lipoprotein lipase in different human subcutaneous adipose tissue regions. Journal of Lipid Research, 32, 423-430.

7. Bachle, L. et al. (2001). The effect of fluid replacement on endurance performance. Journal of Strength and Conditioning Research, 15, 2, 217-224.

8. Ballantyne, C. S. et al. (2000). The acute effects of androstenedione supplementation in healthy young males. Canadian Journal of Applied Physiology, 25, 1, 68-78.

9. Ballor, D. L. et al. (1994). Exercise training enhances fat-free mass preservation during diet-induced weight loss: a meta-analytical finding. International Journal of Obesity, 18, 35-43.

10. Baulieu, E. (1996). Dehydroepiandrosterone (DHEA): A fountain of youth? Journal of Clinical Endocrinology and Metabolism, 81, 9, 3147-3151.

11. Bloomfield, S. A. (1997). Osteoporosis. In: ACSM's Exercise Management for Persons with Chronic Diseases and Disabilities. Human Kinetics.

12. Bonci, L. (2003). Let 'em eat lettuce. Training & Conditioning, 13, 3, 31-36.

13. Brandsch, C. et al. (2002). Effect of L-carnitine on weight loss and body composition of rats fed a hypocaloric diet. Annals of Nutrition and Metabolism, 46, 5,205-210.

14. Brownell, K. D. et al. (1986). The effects of repeated cycles of weight loss and regain in rats. Physiology and Behavior, 35, 459-465.

15. Casa, J. et al. (2000). Journal of Athletic Training, 35, 2, 212-224.

16. Cerny,F. J. Burton, H.W. (2001). Exercise Physiology for Health Care Professionals, Human Kinetics.

17. Clark, N. (2001). Nutrition in Action: How to Fuel Your Body for Sports & Health. A PowerPoint presentation. Human Kinetics.

18. Clarkson, P. (2001). Supplements containing ephedrine: are they safe and do they work? Gatorade Sports Science Institute. http://www.gssiweb.com/

19. da Camara, C. C. (1998). Glucosamine sulfate for osteoarthritis. Annals of Pharmacotherapy, 32, 580-587.

20. DeGroot, L. J. (1995). Endocrinology, 3rd edition. Volume 3. W.B. Saunders.

21. Dolins, K. R. (2002). Sports nutrition for the endurance athlete. Presented at: Inside the Athlete: Fueling the Athlete for Health and Performance. Gatorade Sports Science Institute, October 19, 2002, Philadelphia, Pa.

22. Engles, H. J., et al. (2001). Effects of ginseng supplementation on supramaximal exercise performance and short-term recovery. Journal of Strength and Conditioning Research, 15, 3, 290-295.

23. Engels, H. J. et al. (1997). No ergogenic effects of ginseng (Panax ginseng) during graded maximal aerobic exercise. Journal of the American Dietetic Association, 97, 10, 1110-1115.

24. Gibala, M. J. et al. (2000). Amino acids, proteins and exercise performance. Sports science exchange roundtable 42, volume 11, # 2. Gatorade Sports Science Institute. http://www.gssiweb.com

25. Grant K. E., Chandler R. M., Castle A. L., Ivy J. L. (1997). Chromium and exercise training: effect

on obese women. Medicine and Science in Sports and Exercise, 29, 8, 992-998.

26. Groff, J. L., Gropper, S. S., Hunt, S. M. (1995). Advanced Nutrition and Human Metabolism, 2nd edt. West Publishing Company.

27. Heyward, V. (1991). Advanced Fitness Assessment & Exercise Prescription 2nd edt. Human Kinetics.

28. Howley, E. T. & Franks, B. D. (1997). Health Fitness InstructorsHandbook, 3rd edt. Human Kinetics.

29. Jellin, J. M. Betz, F., Hitchens, K. (1999). Natural Medicines Comprehensive Database. Therapeutic Research Faculty.

30. Kleiner, S. (1998). Power Eating. Human Kinetics.

31. Kreider. R. B. (1999). Dietary supplements and the promotion of muscle growth with resistance exercise. Sports Medicine, 27, 2, 97-110.

32. Kundrat, S. (2002). Nutritional nuances for athletes in stop-and-go sports. Presented at: Inside the Athlete: Fueling the Athlete for Health and Performance. Gatorade Sports Science Institute, October 19, 2002, Philadelphia, Pa.

33. Lockner D.W. et al. (2000). Comparison of air-displacement plethysmography, hydrodensitometry, and dual X-ray absorptiometry for assessing body composition of children 10 to 18 years of age. Annals of the New York Academy of Science, 904, 72-78.

34. Maddalozzo, G. F..et al. (2002). Concurrent validity of the BOD POD and dual energy x-ray absorptiometry techniques for assessing body composition in young women. Journal of the American Dietetic Association, 102,11,1677-1679.

35. Maughan, R. J. Leiper, J. P. (1993). Post exercise dehydration in man. Effects of voluntary intake of four different beverages,. Medicine and Science in Sports and Exercise, 25 (suppl), S2-S10.

36. McArdle, W. D., Katch, F. I., Katch, V. L. (1999). Sport & Exercise Nutrition. Lippincott, Williams & Wilkins.

37. Murray, R. et al. (1999). International Journal of Sports Nutrition, 9, 263-274.

38. Neiman, D. C. (1998). The Exercise Health Connection. Human Kinetics.

39. Nissen, S. K. Abumrad, N. N. (1997). Nutritional role of the leucine metabolite B-hydroxy B-methylbutyrate (HMB). Journal of Nutritional Biochemistry, 8, 300-311.

40. Pieralisi, G., Ripari, P., Vecchiet, L. (1991). Effects of a standardized ginseng extract combined with dimethylaminoethanol bitartrate, vitamins, minerals, and trace elements on physical performance during exercise. Clinical Therapeutics, 13, 3, 373-82.

41. Powers, S. K., Howley, E. T. (1990). Exercise Physiology, 2nd edition Brown & Benchmark.

42. Rankin, J. W. (1997). Glycemic index and exercise metabolism. Sports science exchange #64, volume 10 #1. Gatorade Sports Science Institute http://www.gssiweb.com

43. Rasmussen, B. B. (2000). Androstenedione does not stimulate muscle protein anabolism in young healthy men. Journal of Clinical Endocrinology and Metabolism, 85,1, 55-59.

44. Reimers, K. J. (2001). Glycemic index. Can you use it? Strength and Conditioning Journal, 23, 5,69-70.

45. Reimers, K. J. (1999). High protein diets, right for athletes? Strength and Conditioning Journal, 21, 4. 34-35.

46. Rimm, E.B., et al. (1996). Vegetable, fruit, and cereal fiber intake and risk of coronary heart disease among men. Journal of the American Medical Association, 275, 6, 447-451.

47. Salmeron, J. (1997). Dietary fiber, glycemic load, and risk of non-insulin- dependent diabetes mellitus in women. Journal of the American Medical Association, 277, 6, 472-477.

48. Salonen, J. T. et al. (1992). High stored iron levels are associated with excess risk of myocardial infarction in eastern Finnish men. Circulation, 86, 803-811.

49. Shekelle, P. et al. (2003). The Rand Report. Ephedra and Ephedrine for Weight Loss and Athletic Performance Enhancement: Clinical Efficacy and Side Effects. Evidence Report/Technology Assessment Number 76. AHRQ Publication No. 03-E022.

50. Solomon, P. R., Adams, F., Silver, A., Zimmer, J., DeVeaux, R. (2002). Ginkgo for memory enhancement: a randomized controlled trial. JAMA, 21, 288, 7, 835-40.

51. Tedd, L et al. (1998). Controlling Blood Lipids. Part 1: A practical role for diet and exercise. Physician and Sports Medicine, 26, 10.

52. Tyler, V. (1993). The Honest Herbal. Pharmaceutical Produces Press.

53. Utter, A.C. et al. (2003). Evaluation of air displacement for assessing body composition of collegiate wrestlers. Medicine and Science in Sports and Exercise, 35,3, 500-505.

54. van Dongen M. C., (2000). The efficacy of ginkgo for elderly people with dementia and age-associated memory impairment: new results of a randomized clinical trial. American Geriatric Society, 48, 10, 1183-1194.

55. Vescovi, J. D. et al. (2002). Evaluation of the BOD POD for estimating percent fat in female college athletes. Journal of Strength and Conditioning Research, 16, 4, 599-605.

56. Vescovi, J.D. et al. (2001). Evaluation of the BOD POD for estimating percentage body fat in a heterogeneous group of adult humans. European Journal of Applied Physiology, 85, 3-4, 326-332.

57. Villani, R.G. et al. (2000). L-Carnitine supplementation combined with aerobic training does not promote weight loss in moderately obese women. International Journal of Sports Nutrition and Exercise Metabolism, 10, 2,199-207.

58. Volek, J. S. (1997). Testosterone and cortisol in relationship to dietary nutrients and resistance training. Journal of Applied Physiology, 82, 1, 49-54.

59. Wang, X. D. & Russell, R. M. (1999). Procarcinogenic and anticarcinogenic effects of beta-carotene. Nutritional Reviews. 57, 263-272.

60. Williams, M. (1998). The Ergogenics Edge. Human Kinetics.

61. Williams, M. et al. (1999). Creatine: The Power Supplement. Human Kinetics.

62. Inserra, P. et al. (1999). Immune function in elderly smokers and non-smokers improves during supplementation with fruit and vegetable extracts. Integrative Medicine, 2,1, 3-10.

63. Smith, M. (1999). Supplements with fruit and vegetable extracts may decrease DNA damage in the peripheral lymphocytes of an elderly population. Nutrition Research, 19, 10,1507-1518.

64. Van Duyn et al. (2000). Overview of health benefits of fruit and vegetable consumption for the dietetic professional: selected literature. Journal of the American Dietetic Association, 100, 1511-1521.

65. Wise, J. (1996). Changes in plasma carotenoids, alpha tocopherol and lipid peroxide levels in response to supplementation with concentrated fruit and vegetable extracts: a pilot study. Current Therapeutic Research, 57, 6, 445-461.

66. Shabert JK et al. (1999). Glutamine-antioxidant supplementation increases body cell mass in AIDS patients with weight loss: a randomized, double-blind controlled trial. Nutrition 15,860-864.

67. Tepaske R et al. (2001). Effect of preoperative oral immune-enhancing nutritional supplement on patients at high risk of infection after cardiac surgery: a randomized placebo-controlled trial. Lancet 358,696-701.

68. Hanis T et al. (1989). Effects of dietary trans-fatty acids on reproductive performance of Wistar rats. British Journal of Nutrition, 61,3,519-529.

69. Journal of the American Dietetic Association (2000). Position statement. Nutrition and athletic performance: Position of the American Dietetic Association, Dietitians of Canada, and the American College of Sports Medicine. Journal of the American Dietetic Association, 100, 1543-1556.

70. No authors listed. Glycemic Index: What is It? American Dietetic Association March 19 2004. www.eatright.org/cps/rde/xchg/ada/hs.xsl/home_4456_ENU_HTML.htm (accessed 10/2/05).

71. Hidgon J (2003). Glycemic Index and Glycemic load. Linus Pauling Institute. http://lpi.oregonstate.edu/infocenter/foods/grains/gigl.html (accessed 10/2/05).

72. Martin WF et al. (2005). Dietary protein intake and renal function. Nutrition and Metabolism, Available at Biomed Central http://www.nutritionandmetabolism.com/content/2/1/25 (accessed 10/4/05)

73. Belury M (2002). Beyond the Headlines: Not all trans fatty acids are alike: what consumers may lose when they oversimplify nutrition facts. Journal of the American Dietetic Association, 102,11,1606-1607

74. Shabert JK (1999). Glutamine-antioxidant supplementation increases body cell mass in AIDS patients with weight loss: a randomized, double-blind controlled trial. Nutrition, 15,860-864.

75. Antonio J et al. (2002). The effects of high-dose glutamine ingestion on weightlifting performance. Journal of Strength Condoning Research, 16,157–160.

76. Clark RH et al. (2000). Nutritional treatment for acquired immunodeficiency virus-associated wasting using beta-hydroxy beta-methylbutyrate, glutamine, and arginine: a randomized, double-blind, placebo-controlled study. Journal of Parenteral and Enteral Nutrition, 24,3,133-1339.

77. Miller ER et al. (2005). Meta-analysis: High-dosage vitamin E supplementation may increase all-cause mortality. Annals of Internal Medicine, 142, 60520-60553.

78. No authors listed (Feb 2001). How much protein is enough. Consumer Reports on Health. Consumerreports.org

79. McNaughton LR et al. (1999). Sodium bicarbonate can be used as an ergogenic aid in high-intensity, competitive cycle ergometry of 1 h duration. European Journal of Applied Physiology and Occupational Physiology, 80,1,64-69.

80. Virtamo J et al. (2003). Incidence of cancer and mortality following alpha-tocopherol and beta-carotene supplementation: a postintervention follow-up. JAMA,290,476-485.

81. Davidson G et al. (2005). Influence of acute vitamin C and/or carbohydrate ingestion on hormonal, cytokine and immune responses to prolonged exercise. International Journal of Sport Nutrition and Exercise Metabolism, 15,465-479.

82. Benvenga S et al. (2000). Carnitine is a naturally occurring inhibitor of thyroid hormone nuclear uptake. Thyroid, 10, 1043–1050.

83. Wald DS et al. (2001). Randomized trial of folic acid supplementation and serum homocysteine levels. Archives of Internal Medicine, 161,695-700.

84. Bischoff-Ferrari HA et al. (2004). Effect of Vitamin D on falls: a meta-analysis. JAMA, 291,1999-2006.

85. Boehnke Cet al. (2004). High-dose riboflavin treatment is efficacious in migraine prophylaxis: an open study in a tertiary care centre. European Journal of Neurology, 11,475-477.

86. Garg R (1999). Niacin treatment increases plasma homocyst(e)ine levels. American Heart Journal 138,1082-1087.

87. Cumming RG et al. (2000).Diet and cataract: the Blue Mountains Eye Study. Ophthalmology, 10,450-456.

88. Visalli N et al. (1999). A multi-centre randomized trial of two different doses of nicotinamide in patients with recent-onset type 1 diabetes (the IMDIAB VI). Diabetes/Metabolism Research and Reviews, 15,181-185.

89. Zhao XQ et al. (1993). Effects of intensive lipid-lowering therapy on the coronary arteries of asymptomatic subjects with elevated apolipoprotein B. Circulation, 88,2744-2753.

90. Brown BG (2001). Simvastatin and niacin, antioxidant vitamins, or the combination for the prevention of coronary disease. New England Journal of Medicine, 345,1583-1593..

91. Friso S et al. (2001). Low circulating vitamin B(6) is associated with elevation of the inflammation marker C-reactive protein independently of plasma homocysteine levels. Circulation, 103,2788-2791.

92. Eros E et al. (1998). Epileptogenic activity of folic acid after drug induces SLE (folic acid and epilepsy). European Journal of Obstetrics, Gynecology, and Reproductive Biology, 80,75-77.

93. Sheldon, M (2002). UC Berkeley Wellness Foods A to Z. Rebus.

94. Higdon J (2004). Vitamin C. Linus Pauling Institute. www.lip.origonstate.edu (accessed 4/ 19/05).

95. McAlindon TE et al. (1996). Do antioxidant micronutrients protect against the development and progression of knee osteoarthritis? Arthritis and Rheumatology, 39,648-656.

96. Simon JA et al. (2001). Relation of ascorbic acid to bone mineral density and self-reported fractures among US adults. American Journal of Epidemiology, 154,427-433.

97. Peters EM et al. (2001). Vitamin C supplementation attenuates the increases in circulating cortisol, adrenaline and anti-inflammatory polypeptides following ultramarathon running. International Journal of Sport Nutrition and Exercise Metabolism, 22,537-543.

98. Labriola D et al. (1999). Possible interactions between dietary antioxidants and chemotherapy. Oncology, 13:1003-1008.

99. Iso H et al. (1999). Prospective study of calcium, potassium, and magnesium intake and risk of stroke in women. Stroke, 30,1772-1779.

100. Zemel MB et al. (2004). Calcium and dairy acceleration of weight and fat loss during energy restriction in obese adults. Obesity Research, 12,582-580.

101. Guerrero-Romero F et al. (2004). Oral magnesium supplementation improves insulin sensitivity in non-diabetic subjects with insulin resistance. A double-blind placebo-controlled randomized trial. Diabetes and Metabolism, 30,253-258.

102. Jee SH, Miller ER 3rd, Guallar E, et al. (2002).The effect of magnesium supplementation on blood pressure: a meta-analysis of randomized clinical trials. American Journal of Hypertension, 15,691-696.

103. Guerrero-Romero F (2002). Relationship between serum magnesium levels and C-reactive protein concentration, in non-diabetic, non-hypertensive obese subjects. International Journal of Obesity and Related Metabolic Disorders, 26,469-474.

104. Dobson AW (2004). Manganese neurotoxicity. Annals of the New York Academy of Sciences, 1012,115-128.

105. Hidgon J (2003). Phosphorus. Linus Pauling Institute. http://lpi.oregonstate.edu/infocenter/minerals/phosphorus/index.html (accessed 10/28/05)

106. Hidgon J (2003). Potassium. Linus Pauling Institute. http://lpi.oregonstate.edu/infocenter/minerals/potassium/index.html (accessed 10/28/05).

107. Food and Nutrition Board, Institute of Medicine. Dietary Reference Intakes for Vitamin C, Vitamin E, Selenium, and Carotenoids. Washington, DC: National Academy Press, 2000. Available at: http://www.nap.edu/books/0309069351/html/

108. Prasad AS et al. (1996). Zinc status and serum testosterone levels of healthy adults. Nutrition, 12,5,344-348.

109. Higdon J (2003). Zinc. Linus Pauling Institute. http://lpi.oregonstate.edu/infocenter/minerals/zinc/index.html (accessed 7/7/05).

110. Ibs HK et al. (2003). Zinc-altered immune function. Journal of Nutrition, 133,1452S-1456S.

111. van Loon LJ et al. (2003). Amino acid ingestion strongly enhances insulin secretion in patients with long-term type 2 diabetes. Diabetes Care, 26,625-630.

112. Stearns, DM et al. (1995), Chromium(III) picolinate produces chromosome damage inChinese hamster ovary cells. FASEB Journal, 9,15,1643-8.

113. Kroboth PD et al. (1999). DHEA and DHEA-S: A review. Journal of Clinical Pharmacology, 39,327-348.

114 Villareal DT et al. (2004). Effect of DHEA on abdominal fat and insulin action in elderly women and men. Journal of the American Medical Association, 292,2243-2248.

115. Benjamin J et al. (2001). A case of cerebral haemorrhage-can Ginkgo biloba be implicated? Journal of Postgraduate Medicine, 77,904,112-113.

116. Richy F et al. (2003). Structural and symptomatic efficacy of glucosamine and chondroitin in knee osteoarthritis: a comprehensive meta-analysis. Archives of Internal Medicine, 163,1514-1522.

117. Panton LB et al. (2000).Nutritional supplementation of the leucine metabolite beta-hydroxy-beta-methylbutyrate (hmb) during resistance training. Nutrition, 16,734-739.

118. Metabolic Technologies homepage http://www.mettechinc.com/ (accessed 3/17/04).

119. Bo-Linn GW et al. (1983). Starch blockers--their effect on calorie absorption from a high-starch meal. New England Journal of Medicine, 307, 23, 1413-1416.

120. Hollenbeck CB et al. (1983). Effects of a commercial starch blocker preparation on carbohydrate digestion and absorption: in vivo and in vitro studies. American Journal of Clinical Nutrition, 38,4, 498-503.

121. Umoren J. et al. (1992). Commercial soybean starch blocker consumption: impact on weight gain and on copper, lead and zinc status of rats. Plant Foods for Human Nutrition, 42, 2, 135-142.

122. Schnirring L (2000). When to suspect muscle dysmorphia. The Physician and Sports Medicine, 28,12, http://www.physsportsmed.com/issues/2000/12_00/news.htm (accessed 11/4/05).

123. Broeder CE (1997). Assessing body composition before and after resistance or endurance training. Medicine and Science in Sports and Exercise, 29,5, 705-712.

124. Foster DG et al. (2003). A randomized trial for a low carbohydrate diet for obesity. New England Journal of Medicine, 348,21,2082-2090.

125. Dansinger DL et al. (2005). Comparison of the Atkins, Ornish, Weight Watchers and Zone diets for weight loss and heart disease risk reduction, Journal of the American Medical Association, 293,43-53.

126. Guyton AC et al. (1996). Textbook of Medical Physiology, 9th edition.

127. Rating the diet books. Center for Science in the Public Interest. May 2000

128. Brown TB (2004). Exertional Rhabdomyolysis. Physician and Sports Medicine 34,4 physsportsmed.com

129. Hultman E et al. (1996). Muscle creatine loading in men. Journal of Applied Physiology, 81,1,232-237.

130. Rawson ES (2004). Effects of repeated creatine supplementation on muscle, plasma, and urine creatine levels. Journal of Strength and Conditioning Research 18,1,162-167.

131. National Heart, Lung, and Blood Institute, National Institutes of Health (2000). The Practical Guide: Identification, Evaluation, and Treatment of Overweight and Obesity in Adults (NIH Publication No. 00-4084). www.nhlbi.nih.gov/guidelines/obesity/prctgd_c.pdf

132. Shai, I et al. (2008). Weight loss with a low carbohydrate, Mediterranean or low fat diet. New England Journal of Medicine, 17,359,229-241.

133. ACSM's Guidelines for Exercise Testing and Prescription, 7th edt. (2006). Lippincott, Williams & Wilkins.

134. Phillips, SM (2007). A critical examination of dietary protein requirements, benefits and excess in athletes. International Journal of Sports Nutrition and Exercise Metabolism, 17,S58-S76.

135. Bjelakovic G et al. (2007). Mortality in randomized trials of antioxidant supplements for primary and secondary prevention: systematic review and meta-analysis. Journal of the American Medical Association, 297, 842-857.

136. Feskanich D et al. (2002). Vitamin A intake and hip fractures among postmenopausal women. Journal of the American Medical Association, 287,47-54.

137. Sano M et al. (1997). A controlled trial of selegiline, alpha-tocopherol, or both as treatment for Alzheimer's disease. The Alzheimer's Disease Cooperative Study. New England Journal of Medicine, 336,1216-1222.

138. Masaki KH et al. (2000). Association of vitamin E and C supplement use with cognitive function and dementia in elderly men. Neurology, 54,1265-1272.

139. Lappe JM et al. (2007). Vitamin D and calcium supplementation reduces cancer risk: results of a randomized trial. American Journal of Clinical Nutrition, 85,1586-1591.

140. Wortsman J et al. (2000). Decreased bioavailability of vitamin D in obesity. American Journal of Clinical Nutrition, 72,690-693.

141. Esmarck B et al. (2001). Timing of postexercise protein intake is important for muscle hypertrophy with resistance training in elderly humans. Journal of Applied Physiology 535,1,301-311

Index

About Joe Cannon

Joe Cannon, MS, is an exercise physiologist, personal trainer and health educator who resides Pennsylvania. He holds an MS degree in Exercise Science and a BS degree in Chemistry & Biology. He is doubly certified by the National Strength & Conditioning Association (NSCA) as a Certified Strength and Conditioning Specialist (CSCS) and as a Personal Trainer (NSCA-CPT). A dynamic and motivational speaker who specializes presenting accurate information in easy to understand terms, Joe has been a member of the AAAI/ISMA education facility since 1995, lecturing on the topics of sports nutrition, supplements health and personal fitness training. As the director of wellness for a health club that ranked among the top 100 of all clubs in the United States, he designed and implemented groundbreaking exercise programs for a diverse range of individuals including seniors as well as those with cancer, osteoporosis, fibromyalgia and developmental disabilities to name a few. Joe has written for several publications including *Today's Dietician, Weightwatchers.com*, Fitness Management and the *Journal of Strength and Conditioning*.

Joe can be reached directly by visiting his website www.Joe-Cannon.com

Other Books by Joe Cannon

1. Personal Fitness Training. Beyond The Basics: The perfect book to help people study and prepare for *any* personal training certification. Joe Cannon reviews not only the essential exercise science topics of personal fitness training, but also how to apply that knowledge to the real world. This book also covers real life issues that fitness professionals encounter each day. Essentially, a college-level textbook that cuts out the technical stuff most trainers don't need while focusing on what they should know, the emphasis of the book is to provide the knowledge to work effectively and safely with people and help trainers outshine their competition. This is the companion book to Nutrition Essentials.

2. Nutritional Supplements: A no-nonsense scientific review of 119 vitamins, minerals, herbs and other supplements. This book cuts through the hype and deciphers what works and what doesn't work as well as providing unbiased information about supplement side effects that most people have ever heard before. An eye-opening must read for everyone in the fitness industry! Easy to read and highly referenced, this book is the culmination of over 12 years of Joe Cannon's study and investigation of dietary supplements.

3. Nutrition Essentials: An information-packed nutrition and sports nutrition guidebook that was designed specifically to address the needs of fitness professionals as well as to help them study and prepare for *any* sports nutrition certification. Nutrition Essentials is the companion text to Joe's book on Personal Fitness Training.

4. Health and Wellness Q & A: This book provides quick and accurate answers to over 135 exercise, nutrition and general health questions that fitness professionals are asked every day. No need to search for the answers to peoples questions anymore. The odds are very good they are right here! This is an e-book that can be downloaded directly from Joe Cannon's website.

For more information or to order any of these books, visit www.Joe-Cannon.com.

Quick Order Form

To contact Joe Cannon:

      Email: JoeCannonMSCSCS@gmail.com
      Website: www.Joe-Cannon.com
      Mail: P.O. Box 297 Folsom PA 19033

To order a book directly, go to www.Joe-Cannon.con. Notification will be sent when your order is received.

To use this form to order, fill out the entire form and mail to P.O. Box 297 Folsom, PA 19033. Notification will be sent when your order is received.

Name:_____

Home Address:_____

City:_____State:_____Zip:_____

Phone number:__(_____)_____

Email address _____

Please send me ($25.95) x _____ copies of Personal Fitness Training
Please send me ($24.95) x_____ copies of Nutrition Essentials
Please send me ($24.95) x_____ copies of Nutritional Supplements
Please send me (23.00) x _____copies of Health and Wellness Q & A (e book)
      *Sales tax: Please add 6.00% for all orders shipped to Pennsylvania addresses

Shipping: For orders shipped within the US, please add $5.00 for the first book and $2.00 each additional book. Shipping within the US is free for orders of 10 or more books. For international orders, add $9.00 for the first book and $5.00 for each additional book.

Total book $_____
Sales tax $_____
Shipping $_____
Total $_____

Payment   Visa   Master Card   Check

Card number_____

Name on card_____Exp. Date._____

Cardholder's signature_____

I authorize Joe Cannon to charge the above credit card account for merchant services in the amount for products purchased, including appropriate tax and shipping.

CPSIA information can be obtained at www.ICGtesting.com
Printed in the USA
LVOW090036040613

336821LV00002B/14/P